A BETTER
LIFE AWAITS

Deb & Vic,
You guys are great!
You don't need this
book! Thanks for
your love & support!

"😊
Sue

A BETTER
LIFE AWAITS

*Baby steps
to health and
happiness*

SUZANNE PANTAZIS

LIFESUCCESS PUBLISHING, LLC
8900 E Pinnacle Peak Road, Suite D240
Scottsdale, AZ. 85255

Telephone:	800.473.7134
Fax:	480.661.1014
E-mail:	admin@lifesuccesspublishing.com
ISBN:	978-1-59930-347-5
Cover:	Lloyd Arbour, LifeSuccess Publishing, LLC
Text:	Lloyd Arbour, LifeSuccess Publishing, LLC
Edit:	Publication Services

COMPANIES, ORGANIZATIONS, INSTITUTIONS, AND INDUSTRY PUBLICATIONS. Quantity discounts are available on bulk purchases of this book for reselling, educational purposes, subscription incentives, gifts, sponsorship, or fundraising. Special books or book excerpts can also be created to fit specific needs such as private labeling with your logo on the cover and a message from a VIP printed inside. For more information, please contact our Special Sales Department at LifeSuccess Publishing, LLC.

DEDICATION

For my boys, Nikolas & Kristofer…. the "Pantastic Duo"

CONTENTS

ACKNOWLEDGMENTS

I would like to acknowledge and thank my family and friends, Mom, Dad, Terri, Toni, Rob, Jacquie, Gilles, Jeanette, Jonas, Chris, Stefanie, Juliette, Ron, Nikolas , Kristofer, Paul & Mary, Ted , Kay, Gen, Joel, James, Gary, Barb, Rachelle, Tara, Stacy & Julie . You have all played a part in the writing of this book, by sharing your friendship, your stories, your insights, your listening skills and your love and encouragement. You have inspired me, in many ways which you may not even realize.

To my little dog "Snickers" who helped give me the courage to finally stand up for myself.

To "My Little Polar Bear" - You have shown me true and unconditional love.

I would like to give a special Thank You to Dee Burks from **TAG** for her tremendous help, guidance, encouragement and sense of humour throughout the process of writing this book.

I would like to acknowledge all of the beautiful overweight people out there, who are looking for a ray of hope and encouragement. I hope you will find it in this book.

CHAPTER 1

–Not Another Diet Plan –

I sat at my kitchen table as the tears streamed down my face. I had just gotten off the bathroom scale and realized that I was 100 pounds overweight. I decided to write an entry in my journal. "How do I start the process of losing 100 pounds?" It seemed like such a daunting task. Was my life over? Was I just destined to be an unhappy, unhealthy, overweight person for the rest of my life? I guess this was the point at which I hit rock bottom. I was so sick and tired of being overweight. I did not want to try another diet. I had tried them all, and although I may have lost weight temporarily, I could never just lose the weight once and for all and keep it off. I was angry. It wasn't fair! Why did I have to deal with this struggle? I just wanted to be normal and enjoy my life like everyone else did. I have always been pretty stubborn and determined about things. On this day, I decided I was going to overcome my life-long struggle with weight, and when I figured it out, I would share my secrets to success with others, so they could achieve what had always eluded me—a normal life and a normal, healthy body. I wanted to lose my weight permanently, and I wanted to be healthy, but most importantly, I wanted to feel happy.

So here I am, years later, happy and excited to share my success story with you. I have lost 101 pounds. I am happy. I am healthy. I did it! I did not use drugs or surgery to accomplish this goal. I changed myself from the inside out. I made permanent lifestyle changes at a slow and steady pace. I know that I have unlocked the secrets to permanent weight loss. I have gotten in tune with my body. I have learned how it works. I changed my way of thinking. I no longer think like a fat person. I have learned to nurture my spirit. I am joyously embracing my life each day and feeling so grateful for my life. I have beaten the battle of the bulge, and now I know that I will positively impact many people who will read this book and realize that whether they want to lose 20 pounds or 200 pounds, they don't have to feel hopeless. There is a solution, and I have found it. And now I want to share with you how I turned my life around, and I hope that you will now find the way to turn your life around also. I realize now that my extra weight was just a symptom of something bigger that was going on within me. I understand now that this is more than just about losing the weight. It is also about becoming happy and about leading a fulfilling life and going after your dreams, no matter how unattainable you think they are. So please: read on with an open mind; perhaps your dreams will come true for you, just as they did for me. Remember that it is never too late to start to have a better life.

As you read this book, I would like you to allow yourself to simply take in the information being presented with an open mind and without putting any pressure on yourself to make any changes in your diet or lifestyle at this time. If you can simply be open to educating yourself, this is a huge step in the right direction.

As a person who has dieted repeatedly, I would always fall into the trap of going from one extreme to the other. I would be extremely strict with myself, and then when I cheated (as I always cheated), I took the all-or-nothing approach. I convinced myself that I'd already blown the diet anyway, so I might as well eat the whole chocolate cake! This would negate any positive results I'd had by being so strict and hard on myself.

I have succeeded in permanently losing my weight by slowly and methodically educating myself and by slowly implementing changes at a pace that I could easily adjust to. The changes have not been just about diet and exercise. I have made changes in the way I think and in the way that I approach life. Making gradual changes that you can live with on a permanent basis is the real key to success. It is not about implementing drastic changes into your life that cannot be maintained on a permanent basis. I recently met a young man who has lost a lot of weight. While I feel happy for him, I am also concerned that he will gain the weight back. He lost his weight by doing a lot of exercise. He goes to the gym every day for two to three hours. I worry that he will not be able to maintain his weight loss because he has only made a change in one area of his life, and it will be hard to maintain the level of exercise he is doing for the rest of his life. I hope he will maintain his loss, but I think for the average person, working out for two to three hours a day, every day, will be hard to maintain for the rest of their lives. When we make changes, we want them to be gradual and permanent. Throughout this book, I will educate you about many things that you could do to change your life, but I really need to emphasize how important it is to not overwhelm yourself by implementing changes too quickly.

I will tell you now that if you do this too quickly, you are probably going to fail. So take it from someone who has been there: simply read this book and take in the information. That is all you need to do at the moment. Once you have absorbed the information, you can, if you are ready, begin to implement small changes that will start you on the road to permanent weight loss. Success isn't about hitting it out of the ballpark on the first swing. It is about slow progress that lasts. So please, just sit back, relax, take a deep breath, and know that this is the first step toward a better life.

Diet Reruns

How many times have you started a new diet? How many times have you failed? I have to say there were times I felt like I was the ghost of diets past! I'd tried them all—Atkins, Weight Watchers, The Zone, low-fat, low-carb, low-calorie, taking diet pills, drinking diet shakes, the grapefruit diet, and the cabbage soup diet. You name one, and I'd not only tried it, but I'd failed at it. I kept thinking there was something about me that made it impossible to succeed. Maybe I had an under-active thyroid, or maybe I was a genetic anomaly! Perhaps I was big-boned or had a pituitary problem that made me stuff my face with treats. I can even remember watching a show about a woman with a tapeworm that made her lose weight and thinking, *how lucky!* Can you get one of those on the Internet?

I know it sounds ridiculous, but the desperation of being overweight makes you think some pretty crazy things. The great thing about what I learned by finding my own path to weight loss is that it frees you from these distracting and desperate thoughts. It changes the way you see food, and instead of living to eat, as I did for so many years, you can now just eat to live. Putting food in its proper place in your life completely changes the way you perceive the world and what you can accomplish.

As you learn more about my own personal journey and the techniques that helped me, you will understand that everything I'm telling you is true, even if you may not be ready to hear it right now. You will eventually realize that these ideas will unlock the real you that has been pushed aside over the years by the excess weight. I am here to support you, and as someone who has been exactly where you are now, I know it isn't easy to believe that permanent weight loss is possible. But it is possible, so don't give up on yourself, no matter how old you are or how out of shape you are.

I think that once you really understand how to change and apply these principles, you are not going to be the same person. This will transform your life, and it is going to present you with many new and exciting experiences. It may also scare you. We as humans are really attached to the status quo in our lives—even if we are unhappy. We are comfortable with what we know and are quite often resistant to change. For this reason, I encourage you to mentally and emotionally prepare yourself for the changes that are going to happen in your life. I have personally experienced them, and I would like to help you along your journey because I know that this is going to be the most uplifting and exciting journey you will ever take.

The most fabulous aspect of this journey is that you can go at whatever pace you feel comfortable. I encourage you to not try everything at once, so there is no pressure to follow a certain meal plan, count calories, or keep up the points and exchanges. This is a lifestyle change that is an ongoing process, not a pass-or-fail class. There is no failure here. Slip-ups along the way are merely redirection to get on the path that you choose to accomplish your goal of weight loss. Whenever you slip up, it is an opportunity for learning and growth. Just dust yourself off and keep going in the direction of your goal.

Education is a key part of the process because there is always something more to learn about how our bodies work and what makes them function well. Contrary to some diet gurus, we don't exactly know all the reasons for weight gain or what path is optimal for each person to lose weight. Some things that work for some don't work for others. We are constantly learning as a society, and you as an individual must commit to continually learning about yourself and how your body works. This allows you to adjust your activities and habits to create your own lifestyle of health that can be maintained for the rest of your life.

The changes we are going to undertake are going to impact you and the lives of those around you in ways that you never imagined possible. So with an open heart—and with my outstretched hand to guide you—I extend an invitation to you to begin today to move in a direction to start living your life to your fullest potential. Your future self thanks your current self for having the faith and determination to learn what you need to learn and to do the work that you need to do to make your dreams come true.

Body, Mind, and Spirit

If you've struggled with weight for very long, you probably know by now that losing weight isn't just about the weight. If it was, then everyone who lost weight would have kept it off. If the diet industry actually worked on a permanent basis, there would no longer be a need for the diet industry because everyone would be thin and healthy. We know we need food to survive, but we also can use food as an emotional crutch or a salve for a hurting heart. This is what makes permanent weight loss so hard for literally millions of people. The weight may be a symptom of another problem, be it emotional, physical, or spiritual. We are lacking something in our lives, and food becomes the easy comfort.

By addressing how we think and how extra weight affects our thoughts, you will be able to sort through the reasons that you are overweight and confront those issues first. This is one of the major ways that my method is so different. I don't tell you to start tomorrow eating a bowl of oatmeal and counting those calories. I start with looking at how you got here in the first place. Changing your eating habits won't improve your situation until you really understand yourself and why you have trouble losing weight. I want to help you get to the root of the problem and teach you how to fix things permanently. This is not a race to get there the fastest. It is simply about continually moving in the right direction at a pace that works for you. Until you deal with some of the root problems that are keeping you fat, no amount of food restriction or exercise will produce any type of lasting change.

Knowing that there is some evaluating and understanding of self that has to occur before you start relieves that pressure to produce immediately and unchains you from the bathroom scale. I've had a love/hate relationship with the scale for years—almost like a bad love affair! I wanted it to tell me I was successful, thin, and happy, but most days all it did was tell me I was a failure, fat, and lonely. The stress and emotion surrounding stepping on my scale each morning was nothing short of a religious ritual. I would strip down to nothing just on the chance that my shirt or pants weighed thirty pounds, and then slowly step on the scale. The reading on the bathroom scale would often set the tone of my day. If I had lost two pounds, I would go through the day happily. If I had gained two pounds, I would be grumpy and feel depressed and unhappy.

A key component of my long-term success has been learning how to retrain my mind to move away from some of the emotional pain that started my weight gain and toward new habits that have lead to a fulfilling and joyful life. Few books that talk about weight loss also discuss finding joy in your life or nurturing your spirit. This is a program that will teach you how to nurture your spirit and soul and to lead you toward a joyful and fulfilling life. While you need this nurturing, the truth is that you may be out of practice. Yes, it's true! When we stop paying attention to our own need for joy and spiritual fulfillment, it can be hard to get back in the swing of it again. But it is a vital part of long-term success. I frequently talk to people who lost weight and then gained it back, and one of the reasons (among many) that they regained the weight was that they hadn't learned to fill the void in their lives with things that brought them joy and fulfillment.

Are You Ready?

It may sound like a silly question. After all, who wouldn't be ready to lose weight and improve their lives? But it's not that simple. Making a major life and lifestyle change means you have to step out of your comfort zone in all areas of life. Just like losing weight isn't about the pounds, changing your life isn't just about you. It affects everyone around you, and believe it or not, some people in your life now will not be supportive or happy about the change. I think you have to be mentally ready to make a change. I hope that this book will help you get to that place of wanting to make a change for the better.

When I decided to recreate my own life, I was an unhappy person, living a life of drudgery. I thought I had to overcompensate for what I believed was my failures. I was the typical martyr, feeling I had to fix everything and everyone even if it meant that my own wants and needs were pushed aside. I was in an unhappy marriage with few friends and battled constant aches and pains, mood swings, and anxiety. I had both short and more prolonged periods of depression, as I thought I was hopelessly stuck with this life.

When I was 100 pounds overweight, I did not have to worry about how to deal with receiving compliments and/or propositions from the opposite sex—something I hadn't had for years. I was used to dealing with insults and put-downs. Compliments and propositions were unfamiliar to me. I did not know how to handle it at first. My entire lifestyle and attitude changed, but I had to learn to deal with compliments, sexual advances, and interactions with more people as I became significantly more active in sports. My change affected all of my relationships: with co-workers, friends, my spouse, family members, and my children. While we would honestly like to think that we treat everyone equally, the truth is that when you are overweight, people treat you differently.

People assume that you are lazy, needy, and slovenly and have no will power. People immediately judge you based on your appearance. Some may look at you with pity or disdain. Others may simply have no interest in speaking or interacting with you. I bore the brunt of many insults and rude comments. I was teased and ridiculed throughout my childhood. It is hard growing up as an overweight person. It smashes your self-esteem and crushes your spirit. There are some wonderful, beautiful people who are trapped inside their prisons of fat.

Oddly enough, one of the hardest transitions is adjusting to the idea that you are now thin. It is very revealing of how engrained our habits are when you go to a store to pick up a new pair of jeans and immediately look for the plus-size section. There have been many times as I lost weight when someone would pay me a compliment, and I did not know how to accept it. I would usually discount the compliment. I would even look at pictures of myself that showed me as being thin, and I would not connect with the image of myself. That's not me! Do I really look like that? Maybe that photo just makes me look thinner than I think I am. If someone said, "Hello, beautiful," I would not think that they were speaking to me because I was told for years that I was not beautiful. It took a lot of mental and visual reprogramming to help me adjust to my new body image. It is vital to really contemplate how this type of change will impact your life so you can prepare yourself for both the positive and negative incidents you may deal with every day. I have not really touched on the positive aspects of my change, but there have been many. I have a lot more friends, and my life is more active, exciting, and fun. I have learned how to accept a compliment, and I have received many of them. I find that people treat me nicer and smile at me more often than when I was overweight. The first impression that people have of me is more positive. This has helped to improve my self-esteem and confidence. I no longer feel the need to overcompensate for my obesity because I am no longer obese, and I no longer feel deficient in some way.

Relationships

You may be surprised to learn that some of the biggest changes in your life as you lose weight will be the change in your relationships with the people in your life. You have probably heard the saying, "Birds of a feather flock together." Well, this is very true. We tend to associate with those who share our common interests. It is also true that "Misery loves company." We are connected more closely sometimes to those who share our negative habits and outlook.

So what happens if one of the birds changes its feathers or a miserable person starts feeling happy and fulfilled? I think it is important to take a look at the relationships in your life and understand that some of those relationships will not survive your weight loss, so you must be prepared for this. When you start to change, the people around you may encourage you, but some of the people in your life are going to feel uncomfortable with your changes. Some people may try and sabotage your weight loss because they want you to stay the same, even if it is not in your best interest.

My relationships with my children have also changed. I have always spent a great deal of time with my children. I tried to be a very loving and nurturing parent. When I was very overweight, and when I was unaware of how harmful some of my bad eating habits were for my children, I unintentionally taught them some of my bad habits—such as using food as a reward. If my children were well-behaved, I would take them out for a treat. In my mind, I was doing something nice for my children. I would take them out for donuts and ice cream, pick up little candies for them, or buy them pizza. I had learned early in my own childhood that food was love. So I wanted to give my children all the yummy treats that they desired.

Of course, now I see how I was passing on a bad habit. While I have forgiven myself for this, I have also spent countless hours reeducating my children about food and how it impacts their bodies. If I have any advice for parents, it is to not worry about the past or what you may have inadvertently passed on to your children. What matters is that you can still positively impact their lives and their health. So let it go and work on the good. My relationships with my children have changed, but in a good way. Instead of taking them out for donuts, we will go walking, swimming, bowling, camping, shopping, or skiing. I will take them out for dinner at a nice restaurant on occasion and show them how to make the best choices for them. I spend a lot more time than I used to talking with my children and taking an interest in their lives with regard to what they are learning in school, who their friends are, finding out what they are interested in, and encouraging them to enjoy life and all it has to offer. I resist trying to turn them into something that I want them to be, but rather let them become the persons that they want to be and support them with unconditional love.

My relationship with my spouse did not survive my weight loss, and unfortunately, this is a common occurrence for those who lose weight, whether they are male or female. My husband felt much more comfortable and in control when I was overweight. He felt there was no need to worry about other men trying to steal his wife away from him because my weight kept them away. When I was fat, I can say that my life was unfulfilled because I never went out anywhere, I had few friends, and I had no hobbies or outside interests other than gardening and yard work. I would spend many hours housecleaning, doing things for my family, working on the landscaping, managing the finances, working long hours— and eating and eating and eating. I really did not have much going on in my life because I allowed my weight to hold me back from so many things.

As I started to lose weight, I began to take more time for myself. This improved my outlook and helped me to be more positive, and this, in turn, helped my weight loss. I remember saying to myself one day, "How come I can make sure that my family eats properly and exercises, but I don't seem to have any time left to make sure that I take the time to eat properly or exercise?" I decided that if I did not make some changes in my life, I was going to be so unhealthy and unhappy that I was going to die prematurely or become a burden to my family because of my health issues. You may be aware of this type of burden, because there are so many programs on television these days that show the consequences of long-term obesity and how it can make people homebound and helpless. I didn't want to be that way—ever.

When I was overweight, I was diagnosed as having fibromyalgia—a chronic pain syndrome. I also had high blood pressure, arthritis pain, joint pain, and fatigue and was suffering from mood swings and depression. I also felt resentful toward my spouse because I seemed to do so much for him and my family, and in comparison, he seemed to do so much less. In reality, I was acting like a martyr. On one hand, doing so much for my family made me feel like my life had purpose. It made me feel like my existence on this earth was valuable because they needed me. I had very low self-esteem, and this made me feel like I was worth something. But at the same time, I felt very resentful for all of the effort that I put into caring for my family when they didn't even seem to notice. Then I would often feel guilty for feeling resentful, so I would end up stuffing that emotion down with food. It was a terrible cycle.

I also spent a lot of time working at my business, because I thought that if I earned lots of money, it would give me an increased sense of self-worth, but all it really did was keep me away from my family, make me tired and cranky, and give me an excuse to stay fat. I can honestly say that there is nothing worse (or more pitiful) than a tired, cranky, fat martyr—but that's what I was. I looked for all these external things that would bring me happiness, yet none of them did. I had to decide that I would commit to changing my life and changing my attitude before I could get rid of the weight.

Making Permanent Changes

The kind of change that is real and lasting requires that you replace bad habits with good ones. This doesn't happen all at once, or overnight; it is a slow, steady process. It is important to remember that you never fail until you admit defeat. This is especially true in weight loss, as there is no failure—only quitting or succeeding. Those are the only two options. You may stumble, and you may backslide, but as long as you are willing to keep moving forward, you will learn from your mistakes, and those mistakes will help you to grow and learn. That is all part of the process of becoming healthy and happy.

In most setbacks, there is an opportunity for growth and learning. Start making it a habit to look for this whenever something appears in your life that initially seems negative. It is an understood fact that in every positive event there is some negative, and in every negative event there is some positive, so look for the positive. I know that being fat was one of the best things that ever happened to me. Because of my struggles in life as a fat person, I have learned a lot, and I will now have an opportunity to help others. I choose to be grateful for all the wonderful lessons I learned, and now I can choose to pass on my good habits to my children and their children. I know what I want out of life and how to get it; for so many years, that was a complete mystery to me.

A BETTER
LIFE AWAITS

Remember that whenever you have regret, it means you have learned something. The negative experience is just giving you the lesson so that you choose differently in the future. When you don't take the time to learn the lesson, you will just keep encountering the negative experience in a more extreme way until the lesson is learned. Even my children are experiencing this in their lives. Because they have changed their eating habits, they tend to have emotional reactions now if they eat foods that are bad for them. My son recently went to a friend's birthday party and gorged himself on cake, cookies, soda—you name it. He came home out of sorts and upset, resulting in an emotional crying spell over nothing. As he and I talked, it became very clear to him that the way he was feeling was directly connected to all the bad food he'd consumed. He realized that when he takes in large amounts of sugar, it affects his mood. It first makes him hyper, and later on, when his blood sugar plummets, he gets very cranky and emotional. I was so happy for him when he became aware of how sugary foods affected him. He learned from the experience and became more aware. It is this type of "aha" moment that can completely change your eating habits and solidify your resolve to change.

Most people don't even think when they pick up something and pop it into their mouth. It's a habit, and we don't realize how strong a pull these habits have. A while back, there was a large pothole at the end of our road. It was there for months, and everyone just swerved around it in order to not damage their cars. They finally fixed it a few weeks ago, yet even today I saw several people swerve, just as if the pothole was still there. This shows how resistant we can be to change—not because we don't want to change, but because we are running on autopilot and rely on our old habits. You have to become aware of what you are eating and why. It is the why that is the real key to change—not the sausage or pork ribs or cheesecake.

Solutions, Not Excuses

I honestly think that at one time in my life, I was the undisputed queen of excuses. Excuses are just a way to justify to yourself why you haven't done something to deal with your weight. It allows you to stay in denial, and it prevents you from actively finding solutions to your problem. If someone would ask me, "If you are unhappy, why don't you try to lose weight?" my response would usually be one of my favorite excuses.

For example: "I've tried everything and nothing works! There must be something wrong with me."

Yes, there really was something wrong with me! I had a negative attitude, I had terrible eating habits, I did not realize the impact that some of the foods were having on me, and I hardly ever exercised. I needed to get educated on how to get my health and energy back instead of wasting time feeling sorry for myself.

"I don't have an exercise buddy."

I didn't need another person to exercise. If you decide to have an exercise buddy, don't let that buddy prevent you from going because they don't feel up to it. Make sure you go and do your exercise anyway. Don't rely on someone else to get you moving. Don't let them be your excuse.

"I can't afford it. It's expensive to eat healthy."

Really? How much do you spend on cable and/or Internet services each month? How about on all those snacks, treats, eating out, painkillers, over-the-counter medications such as laxatives, aspirin, pain relief, arthritis relief, sleep aids, cold medicines, prescriptions, and absences from work, not to mention the new wardrobe from changing clothes sizes? I have saved a great deal of money in the long run by eating healthy. I now realize that I can't afford not to eat healthy.

"I don't have time."

What I really didn't have was energy. I felt tired and lethargic, and I wasted a lot of time doing nothing just because I had no energy. I spent countless hours in front of the TV or computer. I spent a lot of time feeling depressed about my weight. I spent a lot more time on doctor visits and feeling sick. I moved a lot slower, and it took me longer to get things done. I now realize that when I eat healthier, I have a lot more energy, and I don't waste time feeling tired and depressed anymore.

"It's not easy being overweight. No one understands what it's like."

What I really should have been thinking is that I don't understand what it is like to be thin and healthy. Instead of feeling sorry for myself that I was carrying around 100 extra pounds, I should have been paying attention to what makes other people thin. What are they doing right? Are you thinking like a victim? Are you thinking "Poor me; I have a lousy life," or "I've tried everything, and I can't lose weight"? If you don't like something in your life, then it's up to you to change it. It is time to stop making excuses and to start looking for solutions to your problems instead.

Find Your Joy

I often tell people to remember that the future-you is so very grateful to the current-you for keeping on track and being brave enough to do whatever it takes to accomplish your goals. I am now my future-me, and when I think back on how far I've come and how hard it was for me to believe that this time I would succeed, I'm incredibly grateful. I'm grateful that I dared to believe in myself and that I dared to start again after so many attempts and so many disappointments.

The joy in my life is beyond anything I dared to hope for back in those long, desperate years, but this joy is here for you as well. Don't worry about the end result right now. Just focus on learning what to do and how to begin your own transformation. A full and beautiful life waits if you have the courage to want it and to simply start by taking one little step at a time.

CHAPTER 2

— Life as a Fat Person —

Fat doesn't just happen. There are many reasons why people become overweight, and it's important to understand what your reasons are so you can address them. This is more than just about diet and exercise. It's about behavior patterns that we have been taught or have fallen into ourselves; often, we are completely unaware of these patterns that keep us fat. We are going to look at ourselves in depth to promote self-education and understanding on many different levels. I would like to ask you to keep an open mind, as it is normal for your mind to resist the idea that you have predictable patterns—but we all do. You may become aware of some behaviors in yourself that you were never aware of before, but please don't let this new awareness cause you any stress or anxiety. Half of the problem is identifying what the problem actually is. You don't have to change anything at this point. You just need to be aware of the issues that are contributing to your weight.

I think that I have a special understanding of what it is like to be overweight, having spent many years being obese. I have experienced things that thin people have never experienced, simply because there are certain issues that you deal with both physically and emotionally when you are overweight that thin people don't have to deal with or even think about.

I know what it feels like to be teased and ridiculed because of my appearance—or even worse, ignored completely. I tolerated being teased as a child, a teenager, and as an adult simply because of being overweight. Since weight is frequently seen as something you do to yourself rather than a disease, teasers somehow feel justified, and overweight victims tell themselves they deserve it, which is not true.

The people who were teasing me often knew nothing about me. They did not know that I was a very gentle and kind person who really just wanted to be normal and have friends and enjoy life. They did not know how intelligent I am. They didn't know that I am a wonderful, loving mother. Most thin people don't know what it is like to have a rash on their inner, upper thighs from their legs rubbing together when they walk. They don't know what it feels like to not be able to shop for clothes in most stores because their sizes did not accommodate anyone my size. They did not feel the embarrassment of having to ask for a seat belt extension when flying because the standard-issue seat belt would not fit around my stomach.

When entering a restaurant, a thin person would not be thinking about where they would have to sit because of their size. I always would avoid sitting at booths, as I often could not fit inside of them. I would look for chairs that were very strong and that did not have side arms, as I could not always fit inside of them and did not want the embarrassment of breaking a flimsy chair. When I would fly on an airplane or ride on a bus, I would always hope that the seat next to me would be empty, as I was too large to comfortably fit into an average airline seat and hated that I might make someone else uncomfortable.

There was also the absolute terror I felt when asked to take my children to the beach or to a public swimming pool. Although I loved swimming and going to the beach, I was so self-conscious of even wearing a pair of shorts or a bathing suit in public that

I could not simply enjoy my day at the beach or at a swimming pool. Because my mind was constantly focused on the fact that people were staring at my fat body with disgust, I denied myself the joy of swimming or enjoying a day at the beach. Going to the movies was something I avoided as well, as the seats did not allow the armrests to move, and I would be squished into a seat that was not big enough to support my body. I was uncomfortable, but more than that, the stares and whispers from other people were too much to bear, and no movie was worth that torture.

Almost everyone who is overweight can recall a particularly hurtful incident where their weight was pointed out as unacceptable. For me, this happened in high school when my drama teacher suggested that I should not continue with drama the following year because she felt that I was too fat to fit into any costumes or to take part in plays that did not have roles for fat people. She made this judgment despite the fact that I had achieved an A in her course. It was extremely hurtful to me. Throughout my teens and early twenties, I experienced rejection after rejection from classmates, friends, and strangers. It was like I lived in a different world from anyone else.

Even after I married and had a family, there were many times when my children were in school that I would have liked to have participated in field trips with them. If it involved swimming, bike riding, skiing, or other physical activities, I would have to make up an excuse about why I could not attend. I couldn't tell them that I could not go on the tobogganing trip or ski trip because they don't sell ski pants in my size. The more I felt rejected, the more I turned to my friend and companion, food, for comfort and relief from the pain. I felt alone in this world. No one could see my true beauty inside because it was buried under 100 pounds of fat. But underneath those 100 pounds of fat was a beautiful and intelligent person just waiting to emerge, like a butterfly out of a cocoon. I just couldn't seem to find my way out! I tried everything that came along, and nothing seemed to work. I saw stories about people like me who'd lost the weight, but I just couldn't make it happen for me. I felt desperate and hopeless. I gave up on myself and became quite depressed and lonely. However, like many obese people, I would always put on a happy face and pretend like everything was fine, even though it really wasn't.

Social Stigma

There's no question that being overweight carries a tremendous social stigma in society today. How you look determines how people treat you. I know it shouldn't be that way, but it is. People make snap judgments about the kind of person you are by what they see, and often those first impressions are wrong. On the surface, it appears that this is no way to live your life because of the pain and emotional trauma it causes.

You also tend to be discriminated against in the workplace when you are overweight. If an employer has two employees to choose from for a promotion and they both do the job well, but one of them is attractive, well-groomed, and thin while the other is overweight, neat, and not so attractive, who do you think is going to get the promotion? While the overweight person may actually be the better person for the job, looks do matter. People like to deal with someone who is attractive, even if they may not be quite as efficient as a less attractive person. This affects your opportunities for job advancement as well as your overall income. It is for this reason overweight people tend to earn less than slim people over the course of their careers.

Dating can be a social nightmare for the overweight individual. The thin person is almost always going to be chosen over the overweight person. You could be the nicest person with the greatest personality; however, most of the time, people are drawn to what is attractive to them. This is not meant to say that overweight people are not attractive and deserving of love. But when it comes right down to it, looks matter. I am not saying that this is fair or that I agree with it. It is simply an observation of how we behave as humans.

So let's look at this a little bit deeper. Is it simply about looks, or is it that your looks give an impression about other things about your personality or lifestyle? What sort of impressions do you get of someone that you see who is 80 pounds overweight? Do you think of that person as energetic or lazy? Positive or negative? Independent or needy? Clean or messy? Athletic or a couch potato? Uplifting or depressing? Healthy or unhealthy? Smart or not so smart? Successful or unsuccessful? Do you ever notice how most of the models for television commercials are thin and beautiful? That is not by accident.

If you don't think that you are being discriminated against because you are overweight, think again. I have felt this discrimination for most of my life and know that it exists and is real. It seemed unfair that I was judged by my looks. But it is a reality of human nature. I always felt angry about this reality, and I wanted to change how people reacted to me. I could accomplish so many other things in my life, but I just could not conquer being overweight. I tried every diet out there, to no avail.

I tried taking diet pills, which worked temporarily until I stopped taking them. Once I stopped the pills, I gained all of the weight back, and then some. I would exercise until I hurt myself or pulled a muscle or became so sore that I could barely move. I would starve myself until I couldn't stand it any longer, and then I would binge and gain back all that I had lost. I tried low-fat, low-carb, low calories, the cabbage soup diet, and every other diet gimmick that was out there. While I might get short-term results, nothing ever changed. I always gained back the weight that I lost and then a little bit more. Maybe there really was something the matter with me. Why could everyone else out there achieve a healthy body weight without even really trying? Why did I get the fat genes I'd heard so much about? Why was I born fat? It made me feel so hopeless and lost at times.

I was so disciplined in so many other areas of my life, but I had no control over that Twinkie or donut that was calling my name. I was defenseless against the temptation of ice cream or chocolate. So I went through my life feeling somewhat inadequate because of this inability to conquer fat. I was depressed and upset with myself because I could not seem to accomplish what the majority of the population did effortlessly.

I felt I had to overcompensate for my obesity by being the most efficient worker, the best homemaker, the best daughter, the best and most thoughtful friend. I finally realized that none of that mattered if I could not achieve a healthy weight. I really just got fed up one day, and I decided that I was smart, very smart, and that I was going to make it my life purpose to solve this problem once and for all. I would not give up until I died or became thin. This became my secret life purpose. The good news is that I finally did figure it all out, which is why you are now reading this book. I discovered why those diet plans, pills, and programs weren't working for me and found something that did work. It has now become my life purpose to help others to get educated and to become aware that there is hope to finally overcome their battle with weight, once and for all.

Food for Comfort, Food as Love, Food as a Coping Mechanism (It's not what you are eating; it's what's eating you.)

I believe we often do things unconsciously and are often unaware of the motivation or reasons behind the things that we do. For example, I remember many times when I would be sitting down to eat some of my favorite foods. I would consciously say to myself that I know I should not be eating this food. I know that I am going to regret this later. I knew that the food that I was eating was not good for me and would keep me fat, but I couldn't help myself. It was like I was an alcoholic addicted to liquor. The only difference was that my addiction was to food. I couldn't understand why I had this compulsion when other people didn't.

When I was a little girl, I remember that whenever I hurt myself or felt upset about something, my mom would be quick to ask me if I would like a little treat to help me feel better. I am sure that my mom meant no ill intent to me because she was just trying to find a way to quiet me and calm me down. I would be given a cookie or a piece of candy if I was upset or hurt. I would quickly forget about what made me feel upset and would focus on enjoying my little treat. Unfortunately, this set up a pattern of behavior that continued on into my adult life. I learned to medicate myself with food rather than to express hurt or anger or deal with emotions in a healthy manner.

I had an especially hard time expressing anger. That was something taboo in my family, so I stuffed it down with food and kept those emotions inside. When I started to become a little bit more aware of my tendency to use food as a coping mechanism, I also noticed that, depending on my mood, I would tend to want to eat certain kinds of foods. If I was especially upset or angry about something, I would turn to my "angry" foods. These were chips, hard candies, peanuts, cheese puffs, or other crunchy foods. As I crunched away and stuffed my food down, I was suppressing my anger and rage. I was not consciously aware of what I was doing for quite a long time, but once I realized this was a pattern of behavior, I noticed that it repeated itself frequently.

I noticed that when I was feeling lonely or depressed, I would tend to look for comforting foods, such as macaroni and cheese, toast with jam, ice cream, cookies and milk, and chocolate and other sweets. Food became my friend and comforter.

Food as an Addiction: Carb and Sugar Addiction (Eating Sugary Foods to Give Yourself an Energy Lift)

I used to suffer from numerous mood swings and low-energy periods during the day. I would often crave a little pick-me-up in the late morning or a couple hours after lunch. I would look to food to provide me with a bit of an energy boost. Perhaps a sugary drink, a chocolate bar, or some hard candies would give me an energy boost, or so I thought. I was unaware of the role that sugar was playing in my life. I was unaware of how my blood sugar levels were affecting my moods and my energy levels.

I learned that when I ate a high-carb, high-glycemic food (donuts, cakes, and cookies) that was low in protein, my blood sugar levels would rise very quickly, and then they would plummet very quickly. When my blood sugar levels were on the upswing, I would be silly and overly energetic for a short period of time, as if on a bit of a sugar high. I felt almost drunk, like an alcoholic, depending on how much sugary or high-carb foods I ate. The faster my blood sugar went up, the faster I would crash into a low blood sugar downer once my sugar rush was over. I would suddenly feel very tired and lethargic. I might become moody, emotional, weepy, or easily agitated when my blood sugar levels would crash.

I thought that there was something emotionally wrong with me. How could I be all happy and giddy one moment and then ready to sleep and/or cry the next minute? I would easily lose my temper when I was in a low blood sugar state. And so, of course, when I was feeling low, I would start to crave sugar again. So I would have my little sugary pick-me-up, and I would feel better for a little while. As long as I kept on eating the sugar or high-carb foods, I would be fine, but as soon as I would stop, my blood sugar levels would crash, and I would feel awful again.

I remember that when I was at the office, I would always have a supply of candies, cookies, mints, or other sugary treats in my desk to keep me happy. I would often forget about all the sugary drinks and candies that I would eat during the day, and I would often lament about how I hardly ate anything all day and couldn't understand why I had such a hard time losing weight. So I was riding the sugar roller coaster of incredible highs and extreme crashes repeatedly throughout the day. It was a really scary ride. No wonder I was exhausted at the end of each day.

In time, I learned that if I had some kind of protein at the beginning of each meal or snack, followed with lower-glycemic carbs, my blood sugar levels would rise slowly and then gradually drop. As long as I kept with this type of eating, I could avoid the sugar roller coaster ride that included mood swings, sugar highs, crying, loss of temper, ongoing weight gain, low energy, and many other bad side effects. As much as I love roller coasters in real life, this is one ride that I have learned to avoid. Just becoming aware of the effect that sugar had on me helped me to feel a bit better about myself. There was a real reason for how I felt, and I wasn't emotionally disturbed. Once I understood that this was just a chemical reaction that was happening in my body, the knowledge gave me some control over my moods, my fatigue, and my behavior. This knowledge helped me to not feel so helpless and lost at times.

Benefits of Being Overweight

This may sound a little ridiculous, but we don't do things that don't benefit us in some way. This means that there are reasons or benefits that may help you choose to stay overweight. These are different for each person, and not all overweight people choose to be overweight (or at least they don't consciously choose to be overweight).

A BETTER
LIFE AWAITS

Being overweight gives you an excuse to stay in the shadows. For many obese people, this is a very prominent reason to stay overweight. Being overweight gives them an excuse for not achieving their dreams. "I could have been a successful singer, but I can't break into the business because they want thin and attractive singers." It relieves a bit of pressure on the expectations of others for us. "I didn't get that promotion because I was discriminated against because of my weight."

You also don't have to deal with others trying to approach you for sex as often when you are overweight. We sometimes use our weight as an excuse to not really get out there and face things that we may be uncomfortable facing in life. The weight functions as a cocoon of protection from difficult emotions we don't want to deal with and situations we want to avoid.

A close girlfriend of mine was moderately overweight when she was sexually assaulted. I noticed that shortly after the sexual assault, she gained a very large amount of weight. When we had a chance to talk about it in more depth, she admitted to me that she felt much safer being overweight. She did not have to worry about men wanting to attack her for sex when she was 100 pounds overweight. She viewed her weight as protection from harm. Some people just don't enjoy having sex with their spouses and will gain weight to make themselves less attractive to their spouse. I also believe that when you are married or in a relationship with someone who is not treating you the way that you feel you deserve to be treated, you may feel resentful and not as sexually attracted to your partner when you are upset or angry at that partner. Often, instead of expressing what you are upset or angry about, you will simply withdraw from that partner, and if you are fat and unappealing to your partner, you tend to drive them away by keeping yourself unattractive to them. Here again, fat is functioning as your protector and guardian.

I remember when I was in my early twenties, I got a prescription for diet pills and lost a lot of weight. I remember how uncomfortable I felt with the reaction of the men in my workplace to a new, thinner me. I started getting men propositioning me at work, which was awkward and embarrassing. I even had a supervisor who made very suggestive sexual comments toward me. I was not used to this! I had been overweight most of my life, and I did not know how to handle it. It made me feel very uncomfortable. I also noticed that when I was thin and cute, the men only noticed that I was thin and cute. It made no difference to them if I had a brain; they just saw a body. When I was heavier, I could have an intellectual conversation with men, and they treated me more respectfully with regard to intellectual matters.

Many people with low self-esteem will end up being promiscuous in their search for love and attention. They are looking for love and affection. However, they will seldom find true love and affection by acting promiscuously. When someone is promiscuous, they will often get used for sex and be rejected afterwards. This leads to shame and low self-esteem, which only makes the person crave love and affection in a more desperate manner. Some will just stuff down their shame and low self-esteem with food and build a protective barrier of fat around themselves that helps them to avoid being sexually attractive to others, which in turn leads to less promiscuity and shame.

What Example Are You Setting for Your Children?

What are you teaching your children by your lifestyle choices? Are you teaching your children how to medicate themselves with food, or are you teaching them that food is simply fuel for your body? It is important to let your children know that the right combinations of food will allow their body to run at its optimum level for energy, health, and wellness. No one wants to pass on unhealthy behaviors, and you can choose to break that cycle.

Are you the parent who shows your child how to lead an active and healthy lifestyle? Or are you the parent that is teaching your child that food is a reward or who views sugary, high-fat foods as treats? Are you teaching your child unhealthy eating habits or healthy ones? Remember that we learn what we live. I lived with a food-reward system as a child, and therefore that's how I was raising my children, too. I think that there are so many people out there who think that fat is something that is genetic. However, I think it is more an indication of what you have learned from your parents with regard to how to cook, how to spend your time, how to feel good or bad about ourselves, and how you are going to relate to food.

You are the product of what you have learned growing up and from the person who fed you for all the years you were a child. This doesn't mean that obesity is inevitable for you or your children. You can choose to reeducate yourself and your children, and to have a different view about food, exercise, self-esteem, health, and lifestyle. Here again, this isn't just some advice I'm handing out. I've lived it. My children have made the journey of learning about food and how it affects the body with me. They no longer see food as a reward, but merely something to be consumed for their bodies to work efficiently. They know that food is for nutrition and that they need to eat a wide variety of foods to get proper nutrition, to feel energetic and healthy, and to look and feel good. If you as the parent choose to change, your children will also follow your example, and everyone will benefit and feel better.

Self-Esteem

Most overweight people will suffer from low self-esteem. They have been hurt or feel insecure and use food as a comfort, which adds weight. Once they are overweight, they will then tend to be teased, rejected, ridiculed, and put down because of their weight, producing a vicious cycle. They are usually the last ones to be chosen for sports teams or even as friends. Healthy and active people like to get out and do healthy and active sports and other activities, and if you are not in shape to take part in these activities, people are not going to invite you to do them, so you tend to get left behind and feel rejected. Self-esteem is very hard to restore when you are overweight and subject to constant teasing and ridicule. It takes a lot of inner work and positive self-talk and positive visualization to regain healthy self-esteem.

Digestive Problems

If your digestive system is not working at its best, you are going to have problems losing weight. There are many things that can cause your digestive system not to work properly. If you have been eating the typical SAD (Standard American Diet), you are probably going to end up with some digestive problems that will further contribute to your obesity. This diet consists of too much fast food and overly processed foods that contain questionable additives. Ingesting foods that are highly processed and full of chemicals can cause numerous problems with your body's ability to process food. It puts a strain on all of your organs. The liver, kidneys, and pancreas have to work harder to process all of the highly refined foods that are going through your body because they are full of additives, preservatives, hormones, and other harmful chemicals. Many people have food intolerances or food allergies that interfere with digestion. I had my gall bladder removed when I was very young. I have been told by a naturopathic dietician that anyone who does not have a gall bladder should take ox bile to help with digestion. Many obese people will have gall bladder attacks, as I did, and these can be quite serious. More and more young people are having their gall bladders removed as well because they have been raised almost exclusively on a diet of fast food and quickie meals. Problems such as diabetes, which was once only seen in older, obese patients, are now affecting our children and young people as we pass our bad habits on to them.

Large numbers of people suffer from gluten intolerances or have problems digesting dairy products. Whenever you take antibiotics, it destroys healthy bacteria that your body needs to properly digest foods. I would recommend reading and educating yourselves about food intolerances and digestive issues that can be corrected by changing your diet, by taking digestive enzymes, by adding healthy bacteria by supplementing your diet with acidophilus, and by eliminating problem foods from your diet.

It is important to realize that every food, liquid, or drug entering your body causes some kind of chemical reaction inside of you, and you need to understand and learn how to create the best possible chemical reactions in your body by choosing what you put into it.

How Are You Spending Your Time?

How do you normally spend your time? Do you spend hours in front of the television? How much time do you spend doing fun things or getting outside and being active? How much time do you spend meditating, nurturing your spirit, or trying to visualize a healthy body image? I know that when you are overweight, exercise can seem like torture. But once you learn how to eat better and heal your body, you are going to find that your energy levels are going to increase exponentially, and you will feel like doing more. Your moods will be much more upbeat, and you will feel a lot better about yourself inside and out. Don't get discouraged if you don't have much energy right now. I am going to teach you how to get your energy back, step by step, so that you will no longer view exercise as a chore, and you will want to get off that couch or out of that computer chair. I am going to teach you how to change your mindset and to help you achieve health and wellness and to nurture your spirit. It's a wonderful thing to discover who you really are as a person without all the weight and burden.

What does it take to make you feel happy? Happiness doesn't happen overnight. But feeling happy and feeling good about yourself is a key ingredient to weight loss success. You are what you think. If you think that you can never lose weight, then that is the reality that you are creating for yourself by convincing yourself it is impossible. I want to teach you how to reprogram your core beliefs about what you think is possible. I want you to find the diamond in the rough that lies within you, just waiting to be revealed. If you are willing to believe in yourself, and if you really want things to be different this time, I am here to help you on your journey to achieve permanent weight loss and wellness.

CHAPTER 3

— *Learning to Think Thin* —

Every day, people lose weight—and not just a little, but a lot! But before you know it, they've gained it right back. When I see this happen, it tells me one thing: they haven't made the appropriate mental shift in their thinking for sustainable results. They continue to think and feel like a fat person on the inside, even though they may have lost weight. It is vitally important to readjust your mental image of yourself, *even before you make significant progress*, to match the way you want to look and the way you want to feel. This is the only way to make a permanent change.

I know it may seem like a small thing when compared to the physical task of losing weight, but I cannot emphasize enough how important it is to make this mental shift in your thinking. In fact, I could probably write an entire book just about this subject, but I am going to try and give you the basics for now so you can begin your journey in the best possible way.

I can tell you that after losing 100 pounds, I have had to learn to readjust the way that I see myself and the way that I feel about myself. However, my shift in thinking did not start after I lost the weight. It started before I lost the weight.

In order to achieve your goals, I think it is important for you to be able to clearly visualize yourself as you want to be and to start believing that what you want is actually possible. You have to start to feel and think like a thin person and start getting rid of some of the thought patterns that keep you fat. I think that if you can get an image in your mind about how your life could be different, then that image helps to keep you moving in the right direction to achieve your goal.

I believe that we think our way to happiness, success, and joy. If you believe that you can never lose weight, then it is likely that you will remain fat. If you believe that this time is going to be different and that you are going to overcome your weight problem once and for all and really believe it to be true, then you will likely succeed. I think that when you are intensely focused and you have a clear vision of where you are going, it helps you to give the proper attention and focus needed to achieve your goals. If you can't imagine it in your mind, it is sometimes hard to believe that you can actually accomplish it.

I think it is also very important to keep a positive attitude and not to let yourself get discouraged when you have setbacks. If you approach things with the right mindset, you will be on the right track to achieve your goals.

Your attitudes and beliefs do affect what happens to you in life, whether you want to believe it or not. Everyone likes to be around someone who is happy, funny, cares for others, and is just pleasant to be around. That person is putting out a positive vibration that attracts others to them in a positive manner. Now think about a cranky, crabby, negative person who always seems to think the sky is falling. They are also putting out a vibration, but theirs is negative and repels others. Thinking thin works in the same way.

If you want to become a thin and healthy person, you want to start thinking like a thin and healthy person now. This is easier said than done, especially if you have never had any experience as a thin and healthy person. I am going to try to teach you how to think like a thin person and how to develop a healthy mindset to lose your weight and to keep it off permanently.

When you start to think differently, and when you adopt new ideas and ways of thinking, your old ways of thinking like a fat person will gradually subside, and before you know it, you will be looking, acting, and thinking like a thin person. There are a number of ways in which your thinking will start to change. As you educate yourself more about how your body works, the way in which different foods affect you, and ways to develop a positive outlook on life, the habits and beliefs that you have will gradually start to change. As you work on improving your self-esteem, you will start to feel more confident about yourself. As you step out of your comfort zone, you will have new experiences, meet new friends, and you will learn that permanent weight loss is possible. Over time, you will change the way you think and feel.

In order to make a permanent change in the way your body looks, you also need to change your mental image of how you look and feel about yourself as a person. I would like you to spend as much time as you can to start to feel like a thin person. This takes practice because for a long time, maybe even a lifetime, you may have thought like a fat person. Try to imagine and feel what it is like to be at your goal weight. Think about this in a lot of detail. The more detailed your image, the better. For example, imagine how great it will be to get to the top of a flight of stairs and not feel the least bit winded. What about sliding into a restaurant booth with more than enough room to spare? You may think about what it will be like to wear stylish and fitted clothing or to walk by a mirror and smile at your svelte reflection. Allow those feelings to flow through you. Think about how you will feel physically and emotionally. Will you walk with confidence? Will you have more energy? Will you feel less bloated and more able to move around easily? Will your love life improve? Think about all those health issues that will be improved or will disappear. Imagine you blood pressure lowered, your sugar levels balanced, and your sleep patterns improved. Imagine all of the compliments that you will be receiving as friends and family notice your weight loss. What sort of new activities will you be able to enjoy that you don't currently enjoy? I would have some fun with this and try to develop a picture in your imagination of what you want to manifest into your life.

Many of us who struggle with weight may have a relationship with food that is unhealthy and negative. Many of us use food for comfort or as a coping mechanism. But you can choose to put food in its proper place, and you can choose a healthy and natural relationship rather than a dependent and destructive relationship. Food is for nourishment, not for emotional help. Thin people don't even consider it as an emotional crutch or a way to soothe their emotions. The more you educate yourself about how certain foods affect you physically and emotionally, the easier it will be to create a new and healthy relationship with food.

Food affects every aspect of our lives, from how we move around to how we feel. Food has the power to heal your body or destroy it. As you learn more about how your own body interacts with certain food, you will discover how to choose food that helps you feel your best and keeps your body functioning well. This includes increasing your metabolism to combat fat and balancing your nutrition to feel energetic and strong. When you imagine yourself fit and strong, you will be able to do anything and go anywhere—including some of those places you may never dream of going right now.

This process is the first step to a real life, not the life where you hide or fade into the background while watching everyone else have a social life and have fun. Imagine a life where you are noticed in the most positive way possible. Think of how excited your friends and family will be and how they will act differently toward you. Think of how your confidence and self-esteem will flourish and what a tremendous role model you will be to your children.

I am still amazed at how many people have been motivated by watching me achieve my goals. So it's a natural extension that I want to help as many people as I can, and you will, too. When others see you having success, it motivates them. It gives them hope. You will lead by example. Think of all the times you've sat alone, eating and feeling trapped by your weight. Now is the time to seize the opportunity to change your life and move past those times.

As your mental picture becomes clear of how you want your dream to look and feel, write it down. Write down your goals and your dreams in a journal or on an index card where you can look at your goals often. Take it out several times each day and spend a moment imagining what it will feel like to reach that goal. Visualize it in your mind. Feel it in your heart. This is such a powerful exercise to help you adjust to your changing image.

There are numerous techniques that I used to help me adjust mentally to my new image of myself as a thin person. Here are a few of the techniques that have helped me.

Positive Self-Talk and Visualizations

As I started my process of losing weight, I instituted a nightly routine of positive self-talk and visualization. I would repeat to myself that I am a beautiful person on the inside *and* a beautiful person on the outside. I would visualize myself being happy and healthy. I would try to really feel what it would be like to not have to worry about my weight and to simply go through life enjoying myself and feeling confident in my appearance. I would try to imagine in a lot of detail how it would feel to be thin, happy, and healthy. I imagined the various activities I would take part in, such as shopping for clothes and what size I'd be wearing. I made it my deliberate intention that I would reduce myself to a size 8, which I eventually accomplished. I had the image so clearly impressed in my mind that my subconscious mind had no choice but to adjust my body to match the image that I was impressing upon my mind repeatedly.

I also made it a practice to counter any negative thoughts about myself or negative comments from others by immediately making four positive statements about myself. For example, if I looked into the mirror and felt disappointed when assessing my figure, I might say something like this to myself: "I am a beautiful person on the inside and on the outside. I am like a beautiful butterfly in a cocoon that is waiting to emerge as the beautiful person that I know exists inside of me but has not yet been revealed. I am a good person. I am a wonderful, loving mother." The whole point of this exercise was to counter the negative image and/or statement by focusing on many more positive statements about myself. There are so many other statements and affirmations that I would say to myself to overcome my internal reprogramming, such as:

- **I am an intelligent person, and I will find out the information that I need to help me to become a healthy, thin person.**

- **I am a hard worker, and I am making good progress.**

- **I am proud of myself for making healthy choices. I am moving in the right direction to achieve my goals.**

- **People around me find me to be interesting, happy, uplifting, and healthy. I am a very likable person.**

- **Good things flow to me easily and effortlessly.**

- **There is an abundance of food, and I am directing my body to dispose of excess fat.**

I would visualize the fat cells dissolving and being removed from my body. I even mentally imagined myself delivering an eviction notice to all of the fat cells in my body. I imagined telling them that they were no longer welcome in my body and that they would have to find a new place to live. I visualized them packing their suitcases and leaving my body. These images are very useful in reprogramming your subconscious mind. Your subconscious mind is much more powerful than your conscious mind. It is the part of your mind that handles all bodily functions, such as breathing, the pumping of the heart, and the filtering of unwanted items out of your body through your kidney and liver function. I would also imagine that I was sending a message to each individual cell in my body, giving it the purpose of reducing body fat.

I would impress into my mind that I do not like desserts. I would say that I find them too sweet, and I do not enjoy them. I would also program into my mind that it feels so good to feel energetic and full of life. The more great things that you can think or imagine about yourself or your situation, the better.

We all know that there are so many great benefits of getting healthy, but it also improves your appearance in ways that you don't always think about. Most people focus on the fact that they will lose weight, which will help them to look better. However, when you get healthy, you will notice that your skin will look better. You will have a nicer complexion, and you will get fewer wrinkles, pimples, rashes, and outbreaks of eczema and other annoying skin conditions than you would if you continue to lead an unhealthy lifestyle. I had an annoying rash on my chest for years, and when I stopped eating dairy products, it went away and never came back. I hardly ever get pimples. I believe that I look younger now than I did ten years ago. Since I improved my eating, I find that my nails are stronger, my hair is shinier and healthier looking, I don't have all that sugar in my mouth to rot away my teeth, and the exercise has really helped me to improve my muscle tone, which make me look less flabby and more in shape. Unhealthy eating really takes its toll on your appearance. I think it is helpful to focus on all the positive aspects of leading a healthier lifestyle and to remember these things on the days when your motivation may be lower than on other days. You don't always see these changes right away. They are slow and gradual. However, the healthier you are, the better you will look and feel. You will have a smile on your face more often, and everyone looks better with a smile on their face.

Of course, I knew that I needed to add a little more physical activity to my routine. I remember how difficult it was for me when I first joined a gym, as it is for many people who are overweight. A gym was not a familiar environment to me, as I didn't like to exercise. I didn't know how to use the equipment, and I was in horrible shape. Just walking into the gym was a frightening and intimidating experience. I felt like everyone would be looking at me and thinking that I did not belong because I was not in shape. Still, the image I held in my mind of meeting my goal won over, and I persevered. I would tell myself repeatedly that I am taking steps in the right direction. At least I am here, making an effort to improve my fitness and to become healthier. This is a good thing. People will look at me and say, "Good for her! She is doing something about her obesity, and she should feel good about herself for moving in the right direction."

Before I went to the gym, I would try to have my workout planned in advance so that I would go with a clear image of what work I was going to do that day. I would focus on getting my workout done, and I would put on music that made me feel good as I exercised. Before long, I really began to look forward to the gym experience. I saw improvements in my performance as well, and my clothes began to sag off me. I had more energy and soon felt like I belonged in the gym. I made friends with other members, and they would encourage me. I would also try to encourage others. It felt good as time went on, and people started to really notice the improvements in my appearance. That motivated me even further.

Positive People

I have a "positive people" board, which is full of photographs of people in my life who make me feel uplifted, motivated, and happy. I keep this board posted right on the wall in my work station at my office so I can look at the photos and remember that I am not alone and that there are positive people in my life who love me and want to see me do well. I also have lots of pictures of myself with those people around me. This board makes me feel good, and feeling good is great for weight loss. You want to try and keep yourself in a positive frame of mind at all times. No matter what happens in your life, try to look for the blessings in all things that happen to you. Many times, something negative will happen, but it may turn out to be a blessing for you. I always make it a practice to look for the blessings or the lessons in all situations that might initially seem to be a negative circumstance.

For example, you might be having a really hard time at work. You may hate your job. You may perceive this attitude as being negative. However, if it pushes you to move in a better direction in your life, say by prompting you to get a new job, then it is actually a blessing. We all have an inner voice and guide that tells us when things are going in the right direction or in the wrong direction. Pay attention to your emotions. If something is making you upset or angry, there is something you can do—you can choose to change your direction in life. You can choose to look at things with a positive outlook or a negative outlook. Maybe you don't enjoy your job because you are not feeling challenged enough or are not making enough money. Let this be the catalyst to help you move onto something better. Don't view it as being negative. Just view it as a push from your inner self, which is trying to move you in a better direction.

You will know when things are right because you will feel happy and joyful. So try your best to feel happy and joyful as much as possible, and you will be surprised at what will manifest in your life.

Baby Steps

One of the hardest things for those who have a lot of weight to lose is the fact that the goal seems overwhelming. If you are a size 22, it can be hard to imagine being a size 8. For that reason, I have always made it a practice to lose weight in ten-pound increments. When I lost the ten pounds, I would ease up a little bit and maintain. I would just focus on allowing my body to get comfortable at the new weight for a while. I think that many of us are very impatient and try to rush to get what we want in life. This can lead to disappointment when things don't go as quickly as we might like them to. However, weight loss affects your entire body and health, and I feel it is important to lose your weight at a slow and steady pace.

It takes time for your body to adjust to your new weight. By gradually losing the weight, it is more likely that you will keep it off. How many times have you gone on a drastic diet? I went on crazy diets too numerous to mention. I would go from one extreme of not even thinking or caring what I ate to the other of being so militant that I knew ever single calorie or crumb that passed my lips. We have all done it, and we have all failed by taking this approach. When you lose weight too quickly, it is such a drastic change for your body, your mind, and your spirit that they can't immediately adjust. Physically, you will feel weak and hungry, and your body is likely to go into starvation mode to slow down your metabolism.

It is much better to lose the weight gradually by making small changes in your habits and food choices that are not so drastic. These baby steps help your body to gradually adjust, while healing your digestive system at the same time. Mentally, it is very hard to make drastic changes to any area of your life that you can maintain in the long term—especially your weight. You will likely get discouraged and feel depressed when you eventually blow your extreme diet, as you inevitably will. But in making small changes, you adjust over time while seeing steady progress, which encourages you to keep going. This will keep you in a good frame of mind, making it easier to adjust your mental image to match your changing body.

When I could comfortably eat and maintain my previous weight loss, I could then decide to kick it up a notch and move on to lose the next ten pounds. To do this, I might try to implement another small change. I would replace a bad habit with a good habit. I would organize myself and think ahead so that I would be successful and not easily sabotaged due to a hectic schedule. This helped me to gradually adjust to my weight loss mentally and physically. As I started to lose weight, I kept taking new photographs of myself to help me adjust to my new image. It's funny that since we don't look at ourselves, we don't see the changes in our bodies as we go along so the mind doesn't adjust to the new, slender you. In my photos, I could gradually see the transformation in my appearance. I would post these photos on my positive people board that is at my work station, where I could see them each day. Looking at the new photos of myself helped me to change my internal image to match my external image. It has helped me to mentally readjust my self-image from a very overweight, insecure, and unhappy woman to a thin, healthy, happy, and confident woman.

The Emotion of Food

Many overweight people use food as a coping mechanism for other stressors in their life. This isn't necessarily on purpose. Their subconscious mind has merely learned to view food as comfort or to use it to avoid feeling emotions or thinking about things that they don't know how to deal with. Food can be used to suppress their anger or anxiety. Food becomes their friend. It is very similar to how an alcoholic might use alcohol. The food is just a different substance.

I think it is important to honestly look at your relationship with food to see if you are using food as an emotional Band-Aid. Are you having a hard time standing up for yourself? Does this create anxiety for you? Are you suppressing your anxiety by feeding it with food?

Can you express yourself when you are angry? Many overweight people are doormats, and I've struggled with this in my own life. Often people are too nice for their own good. They let others walk all over them because they don't know how to express themselves without blowing up. They will often want to say no, but will say yes instead. This is something that has been very hard for me to deal with, and many other people experience the same problems.

I had to learn to face what was bothering me. Sometimes I would be very upset about something that my spouse or a co-worker had done or said. Rather than allow myself to feel angry, upset, or disappointed, I would use food for comfort. I was not consciously aware that I was even doing this. If I suddenly got the urge to binge on some of my favorite foods, I would start to make it a point to try and think about what may have prompted this eating binge. I started to write my emotions in a journal so that I could allow myself to feel and express what needed to be expressed. I might not have been able to communicate verbally or tell the person who I was upset with what I was feeling, but at least I became more aware of how I was using food as an emotional crutch or as a way of avoiding uncomfortable feelings. I started to acknowledge those feelings. I started thinking of things that I could do to stand up for myself. I learned to say no.

For many years, I was in an unhappy marriage. I felt unfulfilled, emotionally drained, unhappy, and frustrated. I had tried to discuss these issues with my spouse and deal with the situation, but nothing ever changed. I felt helpless and trapped in my marriage. My spirit was crushed. I could not be myself. I felt that my spouse was emotionally abusive and that he crushed my spirit. He would insult me and be very controlling. I had two small children and did not want to have to deal with splitting up my marriage. I was afraid to upset my children and my family and my husband's family. I felt that if I chose to change my situation, it would be my fault, and I couldn't cope with the guilt. So I used food to comfort myself and to feed my loneliness. I used food to stuff down my anger, my depression, my anxiety, and my low self-esteem.

As with many people, I had learned at a very young age that food was a treat. As a child, if I fell or hurt myself I would be given a piece of candy or dish of ice cream or a little treat to make me feel better. This became an unconscious habit for me that I used even as I grew up to make me feel better. I would have a little treat to feel better. Food was my best friend and my worst enemy. While it comforted me, it also made my waist size increase. I became unhappier because I grew larger and larger. I did not know how to deal with this. When I became aware of what I was doing, soothing my emotions with food, I realized that I was going to have to face my unhappy marriage. I would write down how I felt in my journal. I would think about ways in which I could start making myself feel better that did not involve stuffing myself with food. I took little steps.

I decided that rather than stuffing my emotions down with food, I would allow those emotions to be felt. My emotions were my internal guidance system trying to push me in the direction that I needed to go. I decided to let myself feel that I felt unloved in my marriage. I allowed myself to feel that I was not living my life the way I wanted to live. I allowed myself to feel my depression, my anxiety, and to cry and feel overwhelmed at the prospect of my family being broken apart. I also started doing things that would make me feel good about myself. I would do positive visualizations. I started exercising. I took piano lessons. I would work in my garden. I would take my children swimming. I would do meditation, yoga, and walking. I decided to get a puppy to ease my loneliness and bring some unconditional love into my life. I remember the day that I got my little puppy. I had wanted a Bichon Shih Tzu dog for a very long time, but my husband would never agree to it. I decided one day that I was not going to let him control me anymore. I simply told him that I was going to get my dog. He had a dog, so why shouldn't I have one? I went and picked up my little puppy, and it made me feel very happy. My husband was furious about it. He told me that it was going to be either him or the dog. I told him I chose the dog. He was stunned. I was so happy with myself for getting up enough courage to stand up for myself. About four months later, I finally made the decision to end my marriage. My only regret is that I took so long to deal with this. I could have been so much happier so much sooner if I had only listened to my internal guidance system, my emotions. So keep this in mind. If you feel trapped, just know that there is an escape hatch somewhere. You just have to find your way. Don't be afraid to feel your emotions. After you let your emotions surface, you can move on rather than refusing to face what it is that you really do need to face. Don't let this information cause you any stress or anxiety. You don't have to do anything right this second; just educate yourself. You don't need to change anything until you are ready.

It is also important to understand that you may need to get some help and support to deal with whatever emotions that are weighing on your mind. Overeaters Anonymous is a support group for people who may have problems with food addiction or with an emotional attachment to food. Many employers offer counseling to employees that could be beneficial. You may find it helpful to read more about emotional eating; there are many good books that can help. You may even want to see a counselor to help you deal with issues, and this is a good thing because you will be dealing with the root of the problem, which is vital in order to keep the weight off long-term.

For now, you can simply allow your awareness to increase and know that there are a myriad of options out there when you are ready. Think back on the events of the past weeks, months, or even years to see if you are using food as a coping mechanism or as an emotional crutch. Search for other ways to feel good rather than using food to make yourself feel better. You must nurture your own spirit and find the joy in your life. In the next chapter, I'll show you how to find that joy and have a new outlook on life, no matter what your situation.

CHAPTER 4

—*Looking Within* —

This may be the most difficult—but one of the most important—chapters for you to read in this book. It is also one of the most difficult and most important chapters for me to write. Even though my own journey has been difficult, I made it, and so can you. It gives me great joy to know that I can fill another person's mind and heart with hope. I have taken my journey within, and I have discovered my life purpose and want to encourage you to take your own journey.

Through my process of self-growth and discovery, I found that it was my life's purpose to reach out to others to give them hope and enlightenment. I am here to put out positive ripples into this world, though for many years I had no idea it was even possible. I was lost, unsure of why I was here and what my purpose or my passion in this life might be. You might be feeling the same way right now, just muddling through, and I want to help you awaken your passion, which may be currently lying dormant within you. I want to help you to reconnect and/or find your spirit, your passion, and your joy vibe. If you will be open to taking this journey, it will be the most rewarding and fulfilling journey you will ever take. I can say from having traveled the same road you are now on that it is a life-changing experience.

I realize that this may seem headed in the wrong direction. After all, if you want to lose weight, you have to talk about what you eat and how much exercise you get, right? While those things are factors in weight loss, they are by no means the most important factors. How you feel about yourself and what you think of yourself are vital in determining whether you will lose weight and if you will keep the weight off. While your thoughts and feelings will inevitably vary from my own, they will be similar in certain respects, and I hope what I convey in this chapter will help you to start shifting those thoughts into those that will assist you as you follow you own path.

Do you ever remember a time in your life when you were so happy or inspired or deeply interested in something or someone that food or eating was the furthest thing from your mind? Something that ignited a fire within you that drove you to do things that you thought you could never do? Try to think about this, and you may have to think all the way back to childhood. Perhaps it was a new hobby or interest in something that really got you excited and passionate about life. Perhaps it was a speech or a sermon that ignited a passion within you. Did you ever feel that feeling of invincibility or that feeling that the sky was the limit and that you could truly do anything? Perhaps a teacher filled your mind with hope or inspiration and gave you a moment when you thought that you could become what you truly wanted to become. Were you excited by the thought that you might become a dancer, a singer, a mother, a father, a teacher, a musician, a doctor, an athlete, a comedian, an astronaut, a writer, or an artist? Were you excited to be in love?

Many of us have not had these moments of excited passion for many years. If you have had those moments in your adult life, that is wonderful. Many of those who are overweight, including me, have not had the pleasure of feeling excited and passionate about life for a very long time. Even as far back as early childhood, there have been many naysayers around who were standing by to crush my dreams. And along with crushing my dreams, they were crushing my spirit by telling me to face the fact that I could not do what I was most passionate about. Perhaps you are now one of the naysayers yourself, telling yourself and others that the dream and the passion you were once so excited about is not attainable. Hope is gone; the drudgery of life sets in, and slowly, we give up on ourselves and our dreams. Our once-bright passion fades. When this happens, we often look to other things to lift our spirits or to make us feel alive and passionate.

Discover Your Childlike Perspective

Have you ever watched young children at play? They are free from worry and deeply engrossed in what they are doing. They are not thinking about what time it is or what bills have to be paid. They are not concerned about the future or the past. They are living in the moment. They are passionate about what they are doing in this very moment. They are alive and excited about what they are doing. They are not competitive, they are not judgmental, they are free from worry, they are not concerned about food, they are not concerned about their self-image, and they have no thoughts of self-doubt or self-loathing. They do not know hatred, jealousy, anxiety, worry, or fear. They are not concerned about whether or not they can accomplish what they are doing. They are simply enjoying doing what it is that they are doing in this very moment. They are not worried about what other people are thinking about them. They don't care about it! They are simply enjoying their moment. If they come across something that they can't do, they just move onto something else or go about it another way.

Life is about the journey, not the destination, and children realize that. They are connected with their spirit, their true self, their creativity, their passion, their joy, and their love. If they like something, they are not afraid to acknowledge that they like it. If they don't like something, they freely express that they don't like it. Political correctness never enters the picture. They are in touch with who they are. They say what they mean, and they mean what they say. So what has happened to us along the way? What has crushed our spirit? What has taken away our hopes and dreams? How have we become out of touch with our true selves?

Humans are the only species that is cognizant of our mortality. We are the only species that is critical of ourselves and others. Imagine several deer in the forest or a meadow standing around and eating grass. Suddenly one deer says to the other, "Oh, I can't believe how fat that deer over there is! She has been eating way too much lately. I think she is depressed about the fact that she and her deer lover haven't been getting along lately." Or perhaps their conversation might be an internal one: *I noticed that those other deer over there are looking at me with disdain. I guess I am not a very good deer. I just can't seem to do anything right these days. I wish the other deer would like me, but my hooves are a strange shape, and I just don't have great antlers, so it's no wonder why they don't like me.* If this sounds utterly ridiculous, well, it is. Deer don't think like that. Lucky for them. For some reason, many humans can be very hard on themselves and on others. We feel threatened when someone does better than we do. It makes us feel inadequate. We judge ourselves and others rather than accept ourselves and others the way they are. Perhaps we need to be more like deer.

Many of us are very good at looking at others and seeing their faults. However, it is very difficult to self-reflect and look within to recognize our own faults and shortcomings. It is hard to realize that there are things about ourselves that we don't like, and many of us will do almost anything to avoid self-criticism. It would be wonderful if this didn't matter, if we could just go through life pretending that everything is okay. But it's not okay, and we often self-medicate these deeply personal wounds with food, just as some use alcohol or drugs.

I know that I am a very beautiful person inside. However, there was a time in my life when I really did not like the person that I had become. How and when did that beautiful little girl inside of me disappear and get replaced with an unhappy, overweight woman who was full of pessimism, resentment, disdain, and criticism of self and others? I had become greedy, selfish, and unmotivated, with low self-worth and very little self-esteem. I was not enjoying my life. Something was missing. After years of conditioning by those who criticized me, I learned how to be critical of others. I was taught how to be jealous, mean, and spiteful. I learned how to insult others. I had been hurt and put down, so I also learned how to hurt and put down others. I learned how to fend for myself be greedy, and hoard.

Self-Defense Can Hurt

Deep within myself, I built a wall around my emotions. In order to make myself feel better about myself, I learned how to criticize and insult others, I learned how to be arrogant and think I was better than others. I lost touch with who I really was. I evolved into someone who was not truly me. How did that happen? It happened because I stopped listening to my internal guidance system, and I started listening to the naysayers, soon becoming one of them. I lost touch with who I really and truly was. In my own way, I was trying to make myself feel better by putting others down. By keeping my focus on gossip and criticizing others, I did not have to look at myself. They say that bullies are really very insecure about themselves. Although I was not really a bully, I would keep my focus on others so I did not have to look at myself and realize my disappointments and my failures. I also had a very difficult time expressing my anger. I stuffed all my anger and my disappointment down with food. Food became my friend, or so I thought. Feeding myself with food became an alternative for feeding my soul with passion.

I was no longer living my life with passion, and the beautiful spirit of mine was crushed and full of hopelessness. My life had no purpose or excitement. My life was drudgery. I was unhappy and unfulfilled, angry and frustrated with my life. I had lost my way, and there was no one there to show me how to overcome. Over time, I slowly started to reflect on myself and the person I had become. I decided I didn't like that person and that I had the power to change. I started by forgiving myself and then forgiving others. When I found it hard to forgive sometimes, I tried to remember that life is a journey, and we are continually learning and growing. We all have the ability to change and evolve into something better than what we were in the past. I believe that many of us are wounded and lost, but we all deserve another chance. I had to take a good, hard look within, and while I didn't like what I saw, I knew that life could be better. It is hard to self-reflect and truly be objective about what kind of person you are. Many of us are unaware of the impact we have on others. We may be arrogant or think we are better than someone else. Often, when you are out of control in an area of your own life, you can tend to be very controlling of others, and I found this to be true. Conversely, we may also be doormats for others to use at will and allow them to take advantage of us. I would often be "too nice for my own good," and afterward, I would feel angry and resentful when I was taken advantage of by others. I didn't realize at the time that I was the only one to blame because I allowed others to take advantage of me rather than setting healthy boundaries.

I could not change who I was until I made the decision to take that good, hard look within and honestly face my own shortcomings. As I evaluated myself and my actions, I became aware of things that I had done that I regretted or—more often than not—became aware of things that I regretted that I had not done. However, I also realized that regret is an opportunity for learning, not an opportunity for judgment. I could choose to learn from my mistakes and grow as a person.

I learned how powerful it is to forgive myself and others. I realized that holding on to anger, resentment, negativity, and pessimism took up a lot of my energy. My energy was being wasted by focusing on negative emotions that did not serve me in any way. I suddenly realized how much easier and uplifting it is to be happy, encouraging, positive, and optimistic. I realized that the only person who is responsible for my happiness is … me. It is not about having the perfect family or marriage or career or trying to impress others—it is about feeling good about who I am and worrying about impressing myself. I need to have the right attitude. I need to keep my passion alive. I need to get in touch with my true self and not worry what other people may think about me.

There will always be those who will stand by to criticize and mock me and others, but I say, let the naysayers mock me if they want to because I know what is true and real. They don't know who they are. They are afraid. I have pity for them because they are truly lost themselves, and they have given up on themselves and others. They have not yet made their journey within. They don't yet have the ability to currently see their own potential and/or the potential in others. We all have the power to choose to try and see our potential and the potential in others. As we see that potential, the future vision of ourselves and others is what will carry us to success.

What Do You Currently Believe About Yourself?

Your core beliefs are operating on a subconscious level in your mind at all times. These beliefs were formed as you grew up based on the opinions of others and by the life experiences that you have had. Your core beliefs, also known as your paradigms, are that small voice that you often hear when you are thinking about whether or not something might be possible. These beliefs/paradigms have been long established in your mind, and they are not easily changed. We are often unaware at how powerful these paradigms/beliefs can be at holding you back from what you want in your life. The negative paradigms are the voices that tell you that you can't do it, that you aren't worthy, or maybe that you aren't worthy enough. They tell you that you are not smart enough, not good-looking enough, or not capable. These negative beliefs are preventing you from living up to your true potential. Positive paradigms are your self-confident beliefs that empower you and lead you in the direction of your goals and bring more joy into your life. These beliefs war with one another constantly, and never more so than when you are trying to accomplish a permanent lifestyle change or a goal such as losing weight, becoming healthier, or improving your life.

These beliefs can interfere with the relationships you have with others. They may tell you that the relationship is doomed to fail, so why try? They may tell you to expect the worst and look for something to complain about. The negative beliefs keep you focused on what is wrong and why you can't do it, while the positive beliefs keep you focused on what is right and why you can achieve your goals. The trick is to delete those negative beliefs and replace them with positive and empowering beliefs.

If you imagine your brain is a computer, then the negative paradigms are like viruses that permeate your system and lead you on a self-destructive path. Some of those negative programs that may be running in your subconscious mind could be:

Self-Doubt. This is when you stop yourself from engaging in a conversation or activity because you don't have enough confidence in yourself or in your abilities. Your negative voice might say something like, "You have always been lousy in math; you won't be able to learn how to be an electrician," "There is no point in trying to talk to that person; they would never be interested in getting to know me," or, "I could never run a mile without stopping."

Lack of Vision. This is the paradigm that tells you that if you've never experienced it, then it can't exist in your life. You simply accept second best because that is what you know and that is what your comfort zone is. This self-talk might say, "I don't know what it would be like to have a great relationship with a wonderful woman because I have never had one in my life."

Low Self-Worth. This is extremely damaging, as it convinces you that you will never be good enough and will never fit in, no matter what you do or don't do. It is the idea that everyone else is worth more than you are, and you might say things such as "I am unattractive," "I am too fat," "I am too old," "I am not successful," or "I am a nerd."

Fear of Failure. Fear is a big paradigm for many people. Because overweight people are treated as failures or as less than intelligent, we can start to believe this idea of who we are, and it can make us very fearful of failing and fulfilling those low expectations. This inner voice might say, "I will be safer doing something that I am comfortable with rather than trying something new and challenging that I haven't done before," or "I will look like such an idiot if I try this and fail."

Procrastination. This paradigm prevents you from acting right now. This paradigm can cheat you out of experiences that you may never get the chance at again. You tell yourself that you need to think about it more before you act. You might say, "It's not a good time right now," "I am going to wait until I lose ten pounds before I join the gym," "I am going to wait until I get past this busy time in my life before I go back to school," or "I will start to improve my diet after the weekend."

Limiting Beliefs. The only limits that exist for us are those we place on ourselves. You may have a desire to better your life, but if you believe that it is impossible or that you are destined to have a disappointing lot in life, then you will never get what you want. You may think, "I always date men who treat me poorly," "I always attract losers," or "I have never done well in school."

Excuses. Excuses are an easy way to let ourselves off the hook and not be responsible for what we haven't done or aren't doing. It's easier to think that something isn't possible rather than knowing that you have the power to change things. You may tell yourself, "All the good ones are gone," or "I am too old to meet new people."

Fear/Jealousy. This is a little different from general fear because it is not about being fearful to try new things. This revolves around the fear of losing what you already have and feeds into the controlling nature many people have. You may have said, "I am afraid that if my wife looks too good, she'll leave me for someone else," or "If my children are weak, they will always need me, and that makes me feel useful and worthy."

Addictions. Some people lie to themselves to justify their addiction by telling themselves things like, "I need to drink to calm my nerves because I had a bad day," "I need these drugs to keep my energy levels up or to keep my creativity flowing," "I don't have a problem; I can quit whenever I want to," or, "I did a lot of exercise today. I can eat that chocolate cake because I deserve it for working out so hard."

Dwelling on Past Failures. The past can be very hard to deal with. You must understand that the past has no bearing on the future or on your potential, unless you allow it to. Just because you behaved a certain way or believed a certain idea in the past is no reason you can't change immediately and have a different outcome in the future. You may find yourself thinking, "I have never been able to lose weight," "People just don't seem to like me," or, "I am unlucky in love."

If you mind is a computer, then you need to run regular virus scans to remove these kinds of destructive paradigms from your subconscious mind. Awareness is just the first step. You need to replace those old paradigms with new healthy ones so that they will take over your predominant way of thinking.

There are many new programs that you can install to lead you in the direction of your goals. You can pick and choose your thoughts and reprogram your mind with healthier paradigms, such as the ones listed below:

Clear Vision: I know what I want and I can clearly see it and visualize it.

Gratefulness: I am so happy and grateful for all the great things that I have in my life. I am going to make it a habit of thinking of all the things that I am grateful for.

Self-Confidence: I can do it! I am capable of achieving anything that I set my mind to.

Looking for Solutions Rather than Excuses: I know I've hit this road block, but I can find a way to get around this.

Positive Ripples: I am consciously choosing to create positive ripples in this world. I choose to see the best in others, and I choose to put as many positive ripples out into this world to consciously make the world a better place.

Empowering Statements: I am a beautiful person on the inside and a beautiful person on the outside. I am having a positive impact on this world. I feel confident in my abilities to achieve any goal that I set my mind to.

Action: I am just going to keep taking steps in the direction of my goals and dreams. I don't have to know how I am going to get all the way there. I am simply going to start moving in the direction that I want to go by taking one step at a time.

Love of Life: I am going to enjoy each day of my life as if it was my last. I am grateful for this day, right now. I am not going to waste it. I am going to make it a point to impress myself today by doing something that will make me feel proud of myself and that will move me in the direction of my goals.

Overcoming Addictions: I realize that I don't need my addiction to make me feel happy. I am in control of my life and my body, and I control my life by controlling my mind. I don't need drugs to calm my nerves. I can accomplish that by exercise, meditation, yoga, or simply choosing to calm my mind. I realize that all the creativity that comes out of my mind when I am influenced by drugs was already in my mind. All the drugs did was help me relax enough to tap into the creativity that was already inside of me. I can find other ways to help my creativity flow that are not harmful to me. I don't need to stuff down my emotions by compulsive overeating or using drugs or alcohol. I will simply allow my emotions to surface.

Healthy Attitudes: I enjoy exercising. It is a great way to help me keep in shape. Exercise is fun, helps alleviate stress, and keeps me healthy and strong. I feel so much better when I eat healthy. I realize that when I eat properly, I have more energy, look and feel so good, and don't get tired or grumpy.

Letting Go of the Past: I am not going to let what has happened in the past determine my future. I will learn from the past, and then I will let it go, and I will move forward on a different road. I have taken many paths in my life, but I know which paths do not work for me, so I will try a different path until I find the right one that works for me.

It is vital that you become aware of the little voices that are playing in the background of your mind. As you hear those negative voices in your mind telling you that you can't do something, imagine yourself pushing the delete button, getting rid of that voice and replacing it with a more positive one. You may need to run a few virus scans to get rid of the negative paradigms and learn how to replace those with positive paradigms. This work must be set in motion before you try to focus on losing weight because if it isn't, the negative paradigms will work against you, trying to sabotage your efforts and convince you to quit. Quitting is easy, and your paradigms always want easy. Get your outlook set to a positive mode, and then do some self-evaluating to see where you really are as a person compared to the person you want to be.

Remember that this process is all about the journey. Don't wait until everything is perfect. Perfect never arrives, and that attitude just cheats you out of living life right now. Working on yourself first is critical, and conquering the inner voices that seek to destroy your progress will allow you to move on to the life you desire.

What would happen if you consciously decided that, rather than looking for things to be angry about, you decided to let go of your anger and make it a practice to look for things in your life to be happy about and to be grateful for? Why not make it a habit to look for the best in people rather than the worst? What if you began to expect good things to happen to you, rather than always expecting the worst to happen? I think that if you did this, more good things would start to manifest in your life, which would give you more things to be grateful for, which would lead to more good things happening in your life, and so on.

You may think that you can't affect the way people treat you, but if you think like that, you are mistaken. What would happen if you decided to take a less confrontational and very respectful attitude toward all the people that you came into contact in your life? What would happen if you decided to set healthy boundaries for yourself? As you did this, a level of mutual respect could develop where neither party would try to control or take advantage of the other party. This type of attitude would create fertile ground for the seeds of warm and loving relationships to grow and develop.

When you hear a negative voice in your mind telling you that you can't do something, change the tape and replace the thought with something new. As you step out of your comfort zone and take on new challenges with a positive attitude, you will start to develop new and better opinions of yourself and your abilities. You will start to change your perspective about what you are capable of and what is your potential.

This is such a powerful way to switch your mindset. Keep in mind that these changes will not happen overnight. You need to keep on top of the negative programs that are playing in your mind until they are all replaced with more positive ones. If you struggle with this, you may want to work with a coach or counselor to help you recognize when you get off track and eventually, with repeated practice, the positive paradigms will become you regular way of thinking. Your negative paradigms will start to dissipate, and the positive paradigms will overtake your life, leading you down a path toward more success, better self-esteem, and a happier and healthier life.

CHAPTER 5

—The Importance of Relationships—

No person lives in a vacuum. We are a product and integral part of the people we grew up with and those we now spend our time with. These relationships create the environment we live in every day and have a large impact on how we live. When it comes right down to it, everyone wants to be loved. Our lives are meant to be shared with others. Loving relationships uplift us and make us feel good about ourselves. It is so rewarding to have warm and loving relationships with others, to be able to share our experiences with, to express and receive love and affection, and to enjoy the simplest of pleasures in life. All humans need to be loved and accepted. I believe the old saying is true: "Money can't buy happiness." I believe that warm and loving relationships can bring you so much happiness, and they don't cost a penny.

Many of us are lucky enough to say that we have people in our lives who make us feel loved and appreciated. These are the people in our lives who love us unconditionally and accept us just the way we are, with all of our faults and shortcomings. These people are usually our spouses, parents, children, and our closest friends. We can even have very special relationships with our pets. Our core people are the people who genuinely want the best for us and feel happy to see us do well.

Having said that, many of our relationships with our closest family and friends are not always warm and loving. In fact, many people have had awful relationships with their close family or have had no close relationships at all. This can lead to the person feeling alienated or even picked on. I know a girl from high school whose mother monitored everything the girl ate because she didn't want her daughter getting fat. The daughter was not fat at all, but became completely obsessed with her weight and afraid that her mother wouldn't love her if she gained weight. Our family can be our biggest supporters, but they can also have tremendously detrimental effects on our mindset if we allow them to.

Many people who carry some extra weight have a hard time developing and maintaining those very important relationships. The underlying insecurity and fear of criticism tends to make us shy away from the possibility of rejection. The next step in taking control of your life and eventually your weight is to learn to develop relationships with others who support your goals so you can feel good while making others feel good at the same time.

I think it is important to be aware of the many different kinds of relationships that we have with others. Some people you only know as acquaintances, and others you know very deeply, perhaps since childhood. Since every relationship will have a different comfort level, some of those relationships will be more meaningful than others. But all the relationships we have will have a direct impact on the joy factor in our lives. The more joy in our lives, the better we will feel and function.

We are constantly interacting with other people during the course of our lives. Ask yourself, "How much time do I spend completely alone?" Now really just think about that for a moment and realize that all the time you are not alone, you are interacting with others. Some of those relationships will be ongoing, and other relationships will be a one-time or sporadic occurrence. Just think about all the people who you come into contact with every day. You relate to your spouse or partner, your friends (both male and female), your children, your parents, your siblings, your co-workers, your pets, and anyone else you come into contact with, many of them complete strangers.

Each of these interactions is a combination of our attitude and their attitude interacting. So you can imagine that if I haven't done my self-reflection, and I am still feeling angry and frustrated, interactions with others will go badly. I certainly know this to be true. You must do the internal work on yourself and then evaluate the external relationships you have cultivated in order to find the support you need to meet your goals.

Attracting the Right Relationships

Every time you come into contact with another individual, you have some choices to make. You choose how you will perceive the person who you come into contact with, and you also choose what you will look for in that individual. The most important choice you will make is whether or not you will look at things with a positive attitude or a negative attitude. For that matter, everything that happens in your life allows you to make a positive or a negative choice.

I firmly believe that when you make it a point to have a positive interaction with the person that you are coming into contact with, you will create the types of relationships that we all want. We all want to have warm and loving relationships.

When you look at your current relationships and evaluate what they are based on, you may be surprised. When I was overweight, I didn't have all that many friends. But one of my friends was overweight like me, and we often got together over lunch or a meal of some kind. We would spend a lot of time pigging out with each other. We both loved to eat, and this shared interest was the glue that held us together. We would go for ice cream together, overindulge in sweets and chocolates, or go out to eat at our favorite restaurants. We would often talk about all the reasons why we could not lose weight and that it was just our poor luck of the draw, bad genetics, or whatever. It is very common for someone with a certain issue or habit to naturally gravitate to others with that same issue. I felt that I could relax and be myself around her without judgment because we both had the same problem. It fulfilled my need to be unconditionally accepted—but it ultimately stood in the way of my goals.

When I started to eat healthier, I no longer wanted to go out and eat ice cream and sweets, or overindulge in food . When I started to change, it made her feel uncomfortable. The dynamics of our relationship started to change. I wanted to go to the gym or go out and exercise. I was excited to tell her about how she could change her life also, but she was not interested in that. She wanted to keep on enjoying her sweets and talking about all the excuses for why she was not able to lose weight. When I started to lose weight, we spent less and less time together because we no longer had that desire for food in common. My success made her reflect on her own situation, and it did not make her feel good about herself.

I wanted to help her and tell her all about what I was doing and how good it was making me feel. She was not yet ready to make any changes in her life, so to her, I sounded like a lecture she did not like to hear, so she slowly cut me out of her life. It was quite hurtful because we had been friends for such a long time. But our friendship was based on a relationship about food and eating, along with self-pity and excuses about why it was impossible to lose weight. If my friend had been ready to make some changes in her life, we could have gone through the experience together, grown, and evolved into thin, happy, and healthy people. But I had to go down this path alone because my friend was not ready for me to make this transition. I knew that I had to follow my path, and she had to follow hers.

As I started changing slowly over time, we saw less and less of one another because we had less in common. Eventually we didn't really have a relationship anymore because our friendship had been based on our mutual problems with food.

Though it won't happen all at once, some of your relationships will suffer as you change—but usually they were relationships that weren't uplifting or beneficial to you. As I changed, so did the people that I spend my time with. I started to meet new friends who had similar interests and beliefs. The new friendships were positive and uplifting. Some of my relationships evolved and improved. As friends and family saw how my changes were making me happier and healthier, it motivated some of them to make positive changes in their lives also. So don't be afraid to move on with your life, even if some of your relationships take a beating. You will develop new friendships and perhaps rekindle old relationships, as people enjoy being around a healthier and happier you. If you don't currently have many friends in your life, don't worry, because you can create new friendships. Many people have joined various support groups, health clubs, or other social events to help them form new and positive relationships. You want to try and surround yourself with people who will uplift and motivate you and who enjoy spending time with you doing activities that make you feel good.

Identifying the Good

It's not uncommon for me to come across people who are in perpetually bad relationships. But having had no good ones—or very few good ones—they don't know what to look for or what characteristics might make a relationship better. Knowing what you want is half the battle. These aren't just my observations. I interviewed a number of people, asking them what they considered to be key characteristics in warm and loving relationships or relationships that were uplifting to them in their lives. This is some of the feedback that I received. I think it is worth taking a look at some of these characteristics in a bit more detail:

Mutual Respect

Everyone wants to be treated with respect. Treat others the way you would like to be treated and expect to be treated the same way by them in return. I think it is important to be open-minded and respectful of other people's individual opinions, personal choices, and ideas. You may not necessarily agree with what they say. However, be respectful enough to let them express their views regardless of who they are or what they believe, and expect them to allow you to do the same.

When you are communicating with others, talk to them in a respectful manner. Don't ever attack a person's character or their beliefs. They have the right to be who they want, and they have the right to believe what they want, just as you do. It is never necessary to be disrespectful toward another individual, regardless of who they are or what their opinions might be.

Respect is a two-way street. Often, overweight individuals allow others to be disrespectful to them and put up with more than they would if they felt better about themselves. Having a little extra weight does not make you less of a person, and no one should ever be allowed to treat you as such. It is important to set healthy boundaries in relationships with others so that the person you have the relationship with knows that you expect to be treated with respect. Respecting another person means you treat them as you would expect to be treated. If you like others to be on time, you need to make it a point to be on time. If you want people to treat your home with respect, then you should treat their home with respect. If someone is not treating you or your home or your belongings with respect, it is important to let them know right from the start what is acceptable to you. Communicate honestly and clearly with one another, and you will be surprised at how well your relationships will thrive. You have to communicate what is acceptable and what is not acceptable to you, which allows you to establish healthy boundaries. For example, if someone walks into your home with their muddy boots on and walks across your carpet, you would need to speak up to let them know that this is not tolerated in your home. If someone is always missing appointments with you or not returning your phone calls, then you need to let them know what you expect. When you do this, one of two things will happen. If they value the relationship with you, they will try to respect your boundaries, or they will not respect your boundaries, and you will end the relationship. It is really that simple.

Open and Honest Communication

It is essential to talk clearly, openly, and honestly with others. This sounds simple and obvious to some, but it can be quite hard in a relationship. Don't assume that the other person knows what you are thinking or feeling. Let them know what is on your mind. Speak from the heart. Be honest and real when talking to others. So many relationships have ended because of misunderstandings or incorrect assumptions or because we can't honestly express what we feel.

Expressing anger is sometimes a difficult issue. However, we need to be able to express our beliefs about the things that we don't like in a healthy, nonconfrontational way. Any criticism should be targeted at the behavior rather than a person's character. For example, "I really don't like it when you leave your muddy boots on the carpet because it leaves a big mess," rather than, "You are such an inconsiderate person for leaving your muddy boots on the carpet!" or, "Could you please try to remember to lock the door when you come in at night?" rather than, "How could you be so stupid to leave the door unlocked all night!"

As we become familiar and complacent in a relationship, we often forget common courtesy, and reinstating it begins with you. You can't control another person, but you can control how you respond. Allow others to express their opinions without feeling threatened by what they are saying. You do not have to agree with their opinions; just allow them to be expressed. Allowing others to express their views helps promote understanding. Since stress in a relationship can be a big motivating factor in emotional eating, this has tremendous bearing on your ability to succeed at losing weight.

Unconditional Love

Unconditional love is about loving a person just the way they are, regardless of looks or beliefs. It means being there for a person without passing judgments. It does not mean being a doormat or compromising yourself in any way. It simply means that you love the person without any conditions. If you want your child to become a doctor and instead your child decides to become a dancer, and you are not happy about that decision, you can feel your disappointment, but you don't stop loving your child because they chose a different path. If you don't want someone you love to drink or do drugs, you do not reject them or stop loving them because they are struggling with this. You simply continue to love them without any conditions attached to your love, while not enabling them to continue on with their addiction at the same time. You love them, but not the addiction. You help them, but you don't help them to continue on with their addiction. Likewise, anyone who has struggled with weight in the past deserves unconditional love from their relationships—yet often they don't get it. Just because you gain a few pounds should not change the fact that you should expect unconditional love from your relationships. Having said that, it is also important to remember that we are all responsible for our own happiness. No one else is responsible to make you feel happy.

Trust

Being able to trust another individual helps the relationship to grow strong. It is good to know that the other person is not going to betray your trust with regard to your security, the promises they have made to you, or by keeping your secrets safe. Trust takes a long time to develop. It gets built up over time when you consistently act in a manner that lets the other person know that you will always be there for them. Trust is earned, and if that trust is betrayed, it may be lost forever, or it may take a very long time to rebuild.

For Better or For Worse

It is important to be patient and understanding with one another. We all have our good days and our bad days. If someone is going through a struggle, it is so beneficial to have someone to talk with who can listen and understand without passing judgments. Sometimes, it is as simple as being a good listener to allow a person to vent their stress or anxiety when they are having a hard time dealing with an issue in their life. It is also about being understanding, encouraging, and forgiving if they make a mistake or if they are having a hard time in life.

The Basis is Friendship

The basis of every good relationship is friendship. It is always such a pleasure to share the important things in your life with someone who can laugh and cry with you. Laughter has healing properties and makes everyone feel warm and uplifted. Shared comfort can make the hard times smoother if you have someone to talk to who will listen. I know there are many relationships that have come to a standstill when each person just goes through the motions, but all is not lost. You need a support system as you change your life for the better, so putting some effort into your relationships is good for the long term. Don't take your relationships for granted, or you will likely lose those relationships. Just because you have been with someone for a long time doesn't mean that you can take them for granted. Take time to feel grateful for the wonderful relationships that you have in your life.

Have Some Fun Together

Isn't it great to just let loose and have some fun? Isn't it so much better to have someone to do that with? Laugh together. Go on a fun outing together. Sing if it makes you feel happy. Kick off your shoes and dance with one another. Be romantic. Act ridiculous and silly sometimes and just enjoy being yourself. Be open to trying new things that your friend or partner might want to experience. Life is an adventure; go out and live it! Live now and start feeling that great feeling that adventure brings.

Encouragement

As we move toward our goals and dreams, it is always nice to hear some kind words of encouragement from another. This helps to shift our paradigms when we have someone else who is encouraging and believing in us. Loving relationships are harmonious. There is nobody controlling or manipulating the

SUZANNE
PANTAZIS

other person. Relationships are supposed to be enjoyable, not stressful.

It is fun to do something nice for someone just because you care and equally as fun to have someone do something nice for you. Good relationships are not one-sided and have a balanced amount of give and take.

The above qualities are some of the characteristics of a good relationship. Below are some of the characteristics of a negative relationship. Hopefully, understanding these characteristics will help you to determine which relationships are working for you and which ones aren't. They may help you to improve your relationships or help you to make the decision to end relationships that are not beneficial to you.

The Negative Relationship

While I was going through my own journey of weight loss, I realized that I was in a very negative relationship. Many other people often find themselves in the same situation. In my case, not only was there little encouragement or support, but there was also a lack of unconditional love. I was angry and resentful and probably quite unpleasant to deal with—and this sent my weight soaring as the stress built within me. While I decided that the best course of action for me was to leave that situation, that doesn't mean that it is the right choice for everyone. Here are some of the characteristics of negative relationships:

Lack of Respect and Constant Criticism

Unhealthy relationships are full of disrespect. For example, "I don't care what you want or what you think," "I don't care if I'm wasting your time or your money," or, "It's my way or the highway!" Criticism is usually targeted at the person rather than at the behavior. For example, "You are such an idiot!" "No person would ever love you!" "You are mental!" "You are so fat and ugly," "You never do anything right," or, "How could you be so stupid?" These types of criticism lead to unhealthy paradigms and low self-esteem and affect your beliefs about what you can accomplish.

Manipulation and Controlling Behaviors

In unhealthy relationships, we will often see one (or more) party trying to control or manipulate the other person. For example, "I am going to make this person feel sorry for me, or I am going to make them feel guilty so that they will do what I want them to do. I am going to tell them what to do, rather than letting them do what they would like to do. I feel superior to them, so I will control them and tell them what to do, rather than encourage them to grow and learn on their own." It is interesting that sometimes people with the lowest self-esteem can be the most controlling and manipulative. If you are the controlling and manipulative person in your relationship, you must self-assess and find ways to change. Control and manipulation stem from fear, and this fear can devastate a relationship.

Co-Dependency and Addictions

Co-dependent relationships can be very destructive. They are usually between two people who are both insecure with themselves. There is usually addiction involved in these relationships, which can include food addiction, alcohol or drug addiction, gambling addiction, and sex addiction. Remember that using food as a coping mechanism is a form of addiction. Both parties may have addictions, and the addictions may be different. One of them may use drugs and alcohol, while the other one may shop compulsively, be a workaholic, gamble, or eat compulsively.

Sometimes, the person in this type of relationship is not secure enough to want their partner to do well for themselves, as it makes the other party feel less useful. For example, "I don't want to make her look or feel too good about herself because then she will leave me for someone else." (This is because I feel inadequate about myself.) "If my husband stops drinking, he won't need me anymore, and he will leave me for someone else."

The enabler or the overachiever in these types of relationships likes to be in control and easily manipulates the weaker party, making them feel empowered by this control. However, it is really a relationship of convenience, not a relationship that is uplifting or rewarding to either party. The weaker party usually uses some sort of addictive substance that prevents him or her from becoming more productive in their life. The more the stronger party keeps looking after the weaker party and bailing him or her out of situations, the more inadequate the weaker party feels, which feeds their low self-esteem, contributing to their continued abuse of food, alcohol, drugs, sex, or gambling.

Violence and Abusive Behaviors

One of the more obvious signs of a negative relationship is one that is violent and abusive. It may be physical violence against the other person or violent acts of destructive behaviors, such as breaking things or smashing dishes, etc. There is serious verbal abuse and attacks of a person's character. This is control and manipulation at its worst. Threats are used to control the other person. Violence is used to control the other person. Attacks on a person's character destroy their self-esteem. If you are in this type of relationship, you need to get some help and advice as soon as possible. To find help you can call a Help Line or a counselor, or ask a friend or the police for assistance.

These Boots Were Made for Walkin'

Just as a good relationship can uplift you and make you feel happy, a bad relationship can crush your spirit, cause you enormous amounts of stress, depress you, and make you feel miserable. When is it right to walk away? We each have to individually answer this question. If both parties are committed to making a relationship work, things can turn around. We have to remember that the only person we can change is ourselves. We cannot force someone else to change if they are not ready or willing to make changes in their lives. So we need to start by making changes within ourselves and becoming more aware of how our beliefs and our actions affect the types of relationships we have with others, as this plays a key role in our ability to succeed.

Be Your Authentic Self

We all have an inner voice or an intuitive guidance system that is connected to our true self. So often in life we stop listening to that inner voice. It gets buried beneath our negative paradigms, which prevents us from hearing our inner voice, the voice of truth. That is the voice of our true selves. It is our soul and our spirit. Sometimes our spirit gets crushed and hurt, so it hides away down deep inside of ourselves, afraid to reemerge.

Our emotions are a signal from our inner self trying to guide us on the path that is right for us. Our inner voice lets us know if something feels right or wrong. This voice is trying to lead us on our way to a joyful and meaningful life, though it is sometimes hard to hear that inner voice. It is sometimes uncomfortable to feel the emotions that are trying to surface. For example, there are many women out there who struggle with the issue of whether or not to have children. This is a highly charged, emotional issue. This is an emotional issue that is often stuffed down with food.

Some women desperately want to have children. However, the person they love may not feel the same way. Or the woman may feel very strongly that she does not want to have children, and her husband may very strongly want to have children. We all have to make this decision for ourselves. However, pay close attention to your inner voice on this issue, and be aware of the negative paradigms that may be preventing you from realizing you full joy potential. Meditation and simply allowing ourselves to feel is a good way to get in touch with our true self and to allow our emotions to surface.

We may try to stuff those emotions down with food, alcohol, or drugs. When we stop our addictions and simply allow ourselves to feel, we start getting back in touch with our true selves. Also by ridding ourselves of our negative paradigms, we can start to get back in touch with who we really are and what we truly want out of life and can finally figure out what really matters to us.

When we can really be true to ourselves, this enables us to be true to others, and then the flood gates will open and warm and loving relationships will grow and prosper. It is very hard to take that journey deep inside ourselves and choose to change, but when you take that journey, it is probably the most rewarding journey you will ever take.

A BETTER
LIFE AWAITS

A dream created to halt reality,
No existence of life, death, immortality
So we search for the truth, which is only a lie
We look for the answer, which has no reply

Our souls are withdrawn, mysterious, black like the night
Feelings kept hidden inside the lonely passage of fright.
After keeping our feelings so deep down inside,
A part of our soul has finally died.
Sadness is concealed, along with our hopes and our dreams,
While our sanity is being torn apart by the seams.
The roar of the panther signifies the cry of the lamb,
Calling for someone to just understand.
The lamb is reality; the panther is not what it seems,
Which gives you the answer to repair the seams.

—Suzanne Pantazis

CHAPTER 6

—Getting to Know Your Body—

To maintain a healthy body, it is important to understand some basic principles about how your body works. I think that we all have to be advocates for our own health and take responsibility to find out what makes our bodies function at their best. When your body is operating as efficiently as possible, you are going to feel good. I am a big fan of the saying, "Physician, heal thyself."

If you think about it, the average person relies on the opinion of their doctor to determine what they should do to keep their body healthy. I only see my doctor once or twice a year, and my doctor sees dozens of patients each day and thousands of patients every year. When I do visit the doctor's office, she will typically spend 15 minutes or less with me during my visit. On the other hand, I spend every waking minute of every single day in this body of mine. When you learn to listen to the cues that your body gives you and then apply a little common sense and a little to research your health, you will find that your body will reveal a lot more about your state of health than your doctor will over the course of the year. I am not saying that you should not listen to your doctor, but I am saying that you should educate yourself about how your body works and take responsibility to find what makes you feel better.

I was always under the impression that I had a slow metabolism and that it was my destiny to be overweight. It was my excuse for being overweight. I was convinced there was nothing I could do that would change things. I did not realize how much power I had to control my health, my digestive system, my blood sugar levels, my moods, my metabolism, my blood pressure, and my mental well-being just by learning how certain foods affect me.

While you may be thinking that there is no way you can learn a whole bunch of medical and nutritional info, relax—you don't have to. You are not going to be able to learn everything, but if you start by learning some of the basics, it will definitely help you to make the best choices for you. It's not about the millions of possibilities; it's about making those few small changes in your life that will make a difference. Once again, I would like to remind you that there is no pressure on you at this point to make any changes to your diet. Simply take some time to educate yourself, and in the upcoming chapters I am going to give you some guidelines for taking some baby steps on the road to wellness and weight loss.

I think for every person, there is that moment when reality hits you like a brick. I remember that day when I sat in my kitchen and cried over the fact that I was 100 pounds overweight. Not 80 pounds, or 90, or even 99. I was 100 pounds overweight. We all have certain breaking points and markers in life that force us to look at ourselves and recognize there is an immediate need for change. Unfortunately, most people have to be hit with a major health setback before they will realize how important it is to change the way we look after our bodies. We have all seen the impact of these major health setbacks: the massive strokes and heart attacks, the diabetes diagnosis, sudden blindness, or the cancer diagnosis. I find it amazing how people always think that it can't happen to them before it actually does. Before these major health setbacks, the body would have been giving the person all sorts of signs that things were not right within their body. Some of those signs are fatigue, shortness of breath, increased weight gain, chronic constipation, high blood pressure, pale complexion, popped blood vessels in the skin or in the eyes, mood swings, upset stomach, skin rashes, dizzy spells, bloating, excessive gas, headaches, chest pains, and other aches and pains. So often these signs go ignored until the body will give a huge sign that cannot be ignored.

How would you feel if you woke up this morning and had a massive stroke that left you paralyzed on one side of your body? Or what if you got a diagnosis of terminal cancer? Or perhaps it might be sudden blindness from diabetes or high blood pressure. Or maybe a massive heart attack. All of these major signs can have permanent and debilitating effects on you. It is so much easier to prevent illness rather than deal with the debilitating impacts of a major health setback. If you knew the week before that you were going to have a massive stroke that would leave you paralyzed, would you make a change, or would you sit back and let it happen? This is something to really think about. Once you are paralyzed, you can't go back and change things. Once your body is ravaged with cancer, it is hard to recover. Once you lose your vision, you can't get it back. So just realize that being healthy is more than just looking good. Being healthy allows you to have a better quality of life.

A good friend of mine was teasing me one day about my healthy eating habits. He asked, "So, are you planning to live to 200?" I replied, "No, but I am planning that while I am living, I will be healthy enough to enjoy my life. I don't want to be suffering, bed-ridden, disabled, or unable to do the things that bring joy into my life." I may not have the perfect body, and I may not eat perfectly all the time, but I do realize that I have a lot of power to control my health, and it all starts with educating myself about how my body works and what makes it run the best.

So after I realized that I was 100 pounds overweight, I let myself have a good cry, and then it was as if a light switch was turned on, and I decided that things were going to change. I decided that I was going to figure it out. I was not going to stop or quit. I was going to keep looking for the answers until I figured out what I needed to do to finally lose my weight permanently. I would not give up. I would logically tackle this problem, just like I logically tackled every other problem or challenge that came up in my life. I would proceed to methodically uncover the information and answers that I needed to lose my weight and to become healthy.

In this long quest, I tried many things. Some of them worked, and some of them didn't work. But with each new idea that I tried, I learned something about myself and about my body. So it was a win-win situation for me. Even if what I tried didn't work, at least I learned from the experience of trying. The most important factor was not to become discouraged and to try and view things in a scientific, logical manner. It was like a very challenging puzzle that I was determined to solve.

Once I'd made my decision that I was really going to do this, I dried my eyes and started by thinking about my previous diet experiences. I had tried many countless numbers of diets over the years, so I reviewed each one and asked myself some honest questions:

- **How long was I able to maintain the diet?**
- **How successful was it?**
- **What did I like about it?**
- **What did I not like about it?**
- **How did I feel when I was on the diet? Was I energetic? Tired? Hungry? Happy? Stressed?**
- **Why did the diet eventually fail?**

- What made it succeed?
- Why couldn't I continue on with the diet?
- Was I able to maintain the weight loss when I stopped the diet?
- Was this diet something that I could live with on a permanent basis?

Unfortunately, after I'd reviewed all my past attempts at dieting, I realized that most diets did not work in the long run. I was usually very hungry, irritable, tired, and stressed while following a diet. My ultimate discovery was that dieting was not the way to go—it hadn't worked so far, and 100 extra pounds was pretty strong evidence that it wasn't going to. So now what?

Once I released the idea that the only way to reduce your weight was some kind of deprivation diet, my mind was free to explore what would work. One of the most important things that I discovered on my quest for a solution was that everything I put in my body produced some kind of chemical reaction. I realized that I was in control of which chemical reactions took place, and I wanted to create the best types of chemical reactions in my body.

Blood Sugar Levels and the Glycemic Index

One of the most important things I educated myself about was something called the glycemic index. The glycemic index is a numerical value given to a carbohydrate-rich food based on the average increase in blood sugar levels when that food is consumed. Foods that have a high-glycemic index produce a quick rise in blood sugar followed by a quick plummet in blood sugar. I noticed that when I ate high-glycemic foods, I would get a short burst of energy, and then I would feel like going to sleep about an hour later. Unfortunately, I could not always have a nap an hour after eating, so I would have to continue eating high-glycemic foods to keep my energy level up. These were high-carb and high-sugar foods such as pop, juice, donuts, muffins, and sweets. Most of the high-glycemic foods are highly processed foods. Once I understood which foods made my blood sugar levels rise very rapidly and how this affected me, I also became aware of the foods that allowed my blood sugar levels to rise very slowly and then gradually decrease over several hours. The low-glycemic foods allowed me to keep my energy on an even level for longer periods of time without having to continually snack on something to keep my energy levels up. Lower glycemic foods are not highly processed. They are high in fiber, nutrients, and protein, and they are lower in sugar content. They are foods like lean meats, nuts, vegetables, whole grains, beans and legumes, fresh fruit, soy products, dairy products, and good fats.

I know you might be reading this and thinking, "Well, hello! I've been told all my life that whole grains and vegetables are better for me than donuts!" And it's true. I've heard that since I was a child, too, but what I didn't understand was that it wasn't just about calories. I think many people who are chronic dieters don't understand that cutting calories isn't the priority. The real goal is feeling better, and how food makes you feel is very important.

Fluctuations in my blood sugar levels did not only affect my energy levels. They also affected my moods and, of course, my weight. Learning how to eat in a more balanced way gave me the power to control my moods, my energy levels, my hunger, and my weight.

For me, it all starts with breakfast. If I can get on the right track with breakfast, this will set the right tone for my entire day. In years past, I might grab a cup of coffee and sugary treat to jolt my system into gear. The problem was, it would leave me craving more caffeine and sugar all day long. It would also leave me irritable, cranky, tired, and moody. Now the goal is to prevent myself from having drastic rises and falls in blood sugar levels. When your blood sugar levels rise quickly, they will also drop quickly, and if you happen to be hyper-insulin sensitive, like most overweight people are, your blood sugar levels will drop lower than they were before you ate in the first place.

Insulin is what the body releases to lower a sudden rise in sugar levels in the blood. When you constantly jolt your system with sugar over a long period of time, your body will overproduce insulin, which then causes your blood sugar level to drop to extremely low levels. Many people who are overweight have this same hyper-insulin sensitivity, which means the more high-glycemic foods you eat, the lower your blood sugar levels will drop, so the stronger your cravings for sweets will be and the hungrier you will feel. This hunger is very difficult to satisfy despite consuming more food on a more frequent basis.

Insulin sensitivity is a precursor to diabetes, which can be deadly. After years of this blood sugar cycle, eventually the body loses its ability to produce insulin at all, and the now-diabetic person must take oral insulin or insulin injections. Diabetics have no ability to lower their own blood sugar, and elevated blood sugar can cause blindness, poor circulation, and organ failure. It can also interfere with the body's ability to heal properly.

Let me give you an example of how I used to eat and how it would make me feel. See if this seems familiar to you.

I would generally be tired and rushing around in the morning, so I would grab something quick and easy to eat. That would usually be some kind of bread product or cereal product (cereal, muffin, pastry, or toast). I would usually wash it down with some kind of juice or a coffee. Another alternative might be a banana or a piece of fruit. In any case, all of my choices were typically very high-glycemic choices. I would usually find that by the time I got to work, I was already feeling kind of hungry again and a little low in energy. So to perk myself up, I would grab a coffee or perhaps another orange juice, and I would have another muffin or pastry at my coffee break.

By the time lunch would roll around, I would be ravenous and would grab some kind of sandwich, a piece of fruit, and perhaps pop or chocolate milk. I could never last until I got home from work to eat, so I would usually eat some chips, a cookie, or some other kind of snack a few hours later. I would always feel so tired an hour or two after lunch, so I would need a little pick-me-up to keep me going until work was done. By the time I got off work, I would need to grab another little pick-me-up for the ride home to tide me over until I could eat dinner. Many times, I would be snacking on crackers, chips, granola bars, yogurt, fruit, or other ready items while I prepared dinner because I was so tired and hungry.

I always felt tired. I also suffered from a lot of mood swings. I was irritable, and I would lose my temper easily. I would suffer from horrible PMS symptoms, gas, bloating, constipation, low energy levels, and unending fatigue. If I tried to go on a diet, I was even more miserable because I would feel hungry all the time. And what about exercise? Are you kidding? That was crazy talk. I was like a walking zombie! All I wanted to do after dinner was to plunk myself down on the couch, snack on my favorite ready-made snacks, and go to bed. That was a typical day in my life.

Once my understanding of how foods affected me changed, I discovered that if I got myself prepared the night before and thought about what foods I could eat to keep my blood sugar levels in a more stable range, then my day went much differently. I realized that I needed to start my day with some kind of protein, along with a balance of lower glycemic carbohydrates. Instead of a muffin and a glass of juice, I might choose two scrambled eggs with a sliced tomato on a piece of whole grain bread with some lettuce and mayonnaise. Instead of coffee or juice, I would have a glass of water. When I ate like this, I found that I functioned so much better when I got to work. I was thinking clearer. I was not hungry. I was productive and would usually work through my coffee break or just have a glass of water.

When lunch came around, I would opt for some kind of protein with salad, and that would keep me feeling satisfied until I got home and made dinner. If I occasionally felt a little hungry before dinner, I would snack on a small handful of nuts or a piece of cheese or a lower glycemic fruit such as an apple. I would keep low-glycemic snacks in my desk and in the glove compartment of my car in case I was running late and needed to eat something. Typically, I have protein bars, Brazil nuts, or pecans. If I was on the run, I would grab a piece of pepperoni, some nuts, cheese, or yogurt.

My main rule of thumb was to eat the protein first and then the carbohydrate. My second rule was to try and keep a rough balance of two grams of protein to every three grams of carbohydrate. You can also add a modest amount of fat to your meal, but try to choose the better fats whenever possible. For a typical meal, I would have 21grams of protein, (which is about three ounces of meat, fish, or eggs) and 28 grams of carbohydrates, which would be comprised of whole grains, fruits, and vegetables, plus my fat, which might be olive oil, salad dressing, avocado, or something similar. (Note: dairy products, soy products, beans, legumes, and nuts contain both protein and carbs, so they will count for both carbs and protein.) Keeping my blood sugar balanced tends to keep my energy levels high, my moods even and stable, and I eat less than I would if I were predominantly eating carbohydrates during the day. With this knowledge, even when I get off track, I know exactly what I need to do to get back on track. If I have a bad meal, the whole day is not shot. I simply make it a point to make the next meal more balanced, and then I will start to feel better.

If I have a very high-glycemic meal and I have the opportunity to sleep, that is what I will do—simply sleep it off or burn it off with exercise. Becoming aware of how your blood sugar levels affect your moods, hunger, cravings for sweets, and energy levels gives you a certain amount of control over those issues. I remember having huge, angry outbursts or mood swings after eating a large volume of sugary foods. This was so out of character for me, and I would feel so out of control. I realize now that it was caused by huge rises and drops in my blood sugar. Once I got my blood sugar under control, I was calm, cool, and collected.

Your Digestive System

Everything we ingest is processed through our digestive system. This allows various nutrients from the foods we eat to nourish and support the body. Our bodies have different digestive enzymes and good bacteria that are needed to break down foods so that the nutrients can be extracted and the waste products eliminated from the body. If your digestive system is working properly, you should be having three bowel movements per day. Most people eating the standard American diet may only have three bowel movements per week, if that. There are many different things that can affect your digestion and cause it to perform poorly, so I am going to mention some of the most important ones.

If you have been eating a lot of processed foods (i.e., fast foods or prepackaged foods), and sugar, drinking alcohol, consuming caffeinated beverages, or have been taking antibiotics, prescription medications, or over-the-counter remedies, it is very likely that your digestive system is not working the way it needs to work. On my journey for answers, I spent a fair amount of time investigating how my digestive system works. I learned about food intolerances (which are different from allergies), parasites, digestive enzymes, and the importance of getting enough fiber and adequate fluids. I also spoke with a naturopathic doctor to learn about colonic cleansing and detox diets and fasts, which were helpful in correcting my digestive system.

Like many people with poor eating habits, I was very often constipated. In the past, I would take laxatives to try to correct this problem, but that was only treating the symptom, not the cause. The reason I was constipated so often was because my digestive system wasn't working properly, and it wasn't working properly because I wasn't eating or drinking properly. I used to drink a lot of black coffee, milk products, and sugary drinks while munching on refined foods with hardly a fruit or vegetable in sight. I had abused my body by eating junk for years, and it had taken its toll on my digestive system. In order to get my health back, I needed to get my digestive system working properly.

Food Allergies and Food Intolerances

Many people have food allergies and/or food intolerances that can lead to weight gain or the inability to digest certain foods. It is very common for people to have a hard time digesting foods with wheat or dairy products. Food intolerances are much different than food allergies. Food intolerances are caused when tiny particles of food get through your intestinal wall and enter your blood stream. When these food particles enter the blood stream, your body thinks that the food particle is an invader, and it takes steps to isolate the particles to prevent it from harming your body. Your body may retain excessive amount of fluids as a way to dilute the effects of the perceived invader. When your body retains fluids, you will have an instant weight gain, and you will feel bloated. Once your body recognizes a certain food as an invader, it remembers that food, and so whenever you eat it, you will have the same symptoms. Food intolerances can be overcome by eliminating the problem foods and by healing your digestive system. Normally, food particles cannot get through the intestinal wall. However, when you eat a lot of refined foods, foods that are full of sugar, caffeine, bad fats, preservatives, and other chemicals, your digestive system gets compromised and doesn't work the way it is supposed to, which can result in food intolerances, auto-immune diseases, cancer, and heart disease. If you suddenly gain a large amount of weight overnight, you may want to start keeping track of what you ate on the day when that happens, as it may be a sign of a food intolerance.

I learned that I had problems digesting dairy products. I discovered this through reading about food intolerances and by listening to my body signals. Whenever I would eat dairy products, I would gain five to eight pounds overnight. I would also get very constipated. I spoke with a naturopath, who explained to me that most people cannot properly digest dairy products. Dairy products come from cow's milk that is designed for a baby cow to digest. Cows have four stomachs to digest their food, whereas humans have only one. This makes it difficult for us to digest milk from a cow because the cow's milk was intended to be consumed by cows, not people.

To be honest, this was something that I did not want to hear. I loved my dairy products: ice cream, cheese, sour cream, milk with cereal, and yogurt. I thought that dairy products were supposed to be good for me. Over time, I learned that there were many other ways to get my calcium, and I was sick and tired of being constipated and overweight, so I decided that I would try to eliminate dairy products from my diet to see what would happen.

After one week of eliminating dairy products, I noticed two things. First of all, I was delighted to lose eight pounds. I also noticed that my nasal passages were no longer congested. This was an unexpected and very pleasant surprise. For years, I had suffered with nasal congestion and lots of phlegm in my throat. I was always taking cold medications and decongestants, but I could never get rid of this congestion. I just got used to it and figured that I must have allergies to dust or various pollens. If you are also suffering from nasal congestion, you may also have some issues with dairy products. After staying away from dairy products for a longer period of time, I noticed that a rash that I had for many years on my chest just went away and never came back.

I now notice that if I get off track and eat dairy products, I will get congested right away, I will also get very bloated, and the constipation sets in very quickly. With the knowledge that I have about how dairy products affect me, it is much easier for me to stay away from these products because it is not worth eating them to end up feeling awful for many days afterward.

You may also have food intolerances. Some of the most common are dairy, wheat, gluten, yeast, and peanuts. Some of the common signs of food intolerances are bloating, excessive gas, constipation, and sudden weight gain. If you suspect that you may have food intolerances, do some more research. I would recommend reading *The Food Intolerance Bible* to get more information on food intolerances and allergies. You can find this book on Amazon.com.

Food intolerances differ from allergies in one key way. Allergies can be life-threatening. Even the hint of certain foods can cause a severe reaction, often requiring immediate medical attention. Intolerances just make you feel bad, which is why they go unnoticed for years by most people. The symptoms are easily attributable to other issues, so you continue to eat the foods that you may love, never knowing they don't love you back.

A very close friend of mine who was very overweight also suffered for years from extremely severe migraine headaches. In an effort to lose weight, she decided to eliminate wheat and dairy products from her diet. She not only lost weight, but also cured herself of her migraine headaches. She had no idea what was causing her migraines, and it was simply by accident that she found out that wheat and dairy products were triggering her migraines.

Another close friend of mine has suffered with nasal congestion and asthma all of his life. I suggested that he should try and eliminate dairy products from his diet. He followed my advice, and in four days, he was completely free from congestion.

Another close friend of mine suffered from gluten intolerance. Whenever he ate foods containing gluten, he would feel sick and bloated. By having the knowledge of how these foods affect them, these people have the power to control their symptoms. This knowledge is power.

My research indicates that a poor diet, food intolerances, and allergies may be responsible, at least in part, for many nonspecific diagnoses and may intensify others, such as chronic fatigue syndrome, multiple sclerosis, rheumatoid arthritis, osteoarthritis, digestive problems, weight gain, diabetes, heart disease, kidney failure, cancer, Crohn's disease, irritable bowel syndrome, and migraine headaches. Start paying attention to how you feel after eating certain foods. Since I have listened to what my body is telling me and have changed the way in which I eat, I no longer suffer from high blood pressure, arthritis, constipation, poor digestion, regular headaches, fibromyalgia, fatigue, insomnia, and obesity. If you don't think that what you are eating may be making you sick, I hope this encourages you to reconsider and start being an advocate for your own health.

It is important to remember that everything that you put in your body impacts your health. Here are a few little interesting tidbits that I learned along the way that may help you to improve your health:

- **Whenever you take antibiotics, it kills the good bacteria in your digestive system. In order to put these good** bacteria back, it is advised to take acidophilus until your digestive system gets back to normal.

- Many overweight people have a problem with their thyroid function, even though the standard blood test will show their thyroid as being normal. Iodine is a key nutrient for proper function of the thyroid. A rich source of iodine is kelp. Many women will have problems with their thyroid as they begin going through menopause. An easy way to see if your thyroid is working properly is by taking your temperature at certain times of the day. For more information on how to do these temperature tests, visit www.stopthethyroidmadness.com.

- In order to fully clean out my digestive system, I went to a clinic and had colonic cleansing done. This is a method in which they fill your bowels with water and then draw the water and fecal matter out. It took several treatments to get things fully cleaned out, but I felt much better afterwards.

- Another way to heal and clean out your digestive system is to try an herbal cleanse, during which you take natural supplements that help you to clean out and detoxify your digestive system. These can be found at many health-food stores.

- Fasting is a good way to occasionally give your digestive system a break. There are many different herbs and natural supplements that you can take while fasting that help your digestive system to heal and rid itself of toxins.

- Some people have low digestive enzymes, which makes it difficult to properly digest foods. You may need to supplement your diet with digestive enzymes.

- Exercise helps with digestion, reduces stress, helps build muscles, and also helps to speed up your metabolism.

- You need to drink at least eight eight-ounce glasses of water per day to provide enough fluids to your body. Whenever I feel myself getting a little constipated, I immediately think about how much water I have been drinking.

- Do you suffer with premenstrual symptoms or perimenopause or menopause symptoms? Did you know that by making changes in your diet, you can reduce or eliminate your symptoms? Foods like sugar, caffeine, and alcohol will make your symptoms worse.

- If you suffer with PMS or menopause, there are many natural remedies that may help to alleviate your symptoms. Some of those natural remedies are evening primrose oil, red clover, maca root, dong quai, and black cohosh. These herbs can help with symptoms such as hot flashes, vaginal dryness, heart palpitations, and poor memory. Most of these herbs can be found at most health-food stores. Women who are suffering from hormonal fluctuations will often benefit from increasing their intake of phytoestrogens in their diet. Phytoestrogens are hormone-like chemicals found in plants such as soy products, wild yam, and ground flax seeds. If you are suffering with hormone fluctuations, changing your diet to increase your phytoestrogens can help. Many woman suffering with PMS, menopause, or perimenopause use wild yam cream or natural progesterone cream to help alleviate their symptoms. Natural progesterone cream is different than synthetic progesterone cream, which has been found to increase your risk of breast cancer. It is a good idea to consult with a naturopathic or medical doctor to have your hormone levels checked to see if you would benefit from some of these natural remedies.

- Did you know that men who drink one glass of soy milk a day have a 70 percent reduced risk of developing prostate cancer?

- Did you know that by eating a small handful of pecans each day, you can reduce your bad cholesterol in your body?

As you can see, there are lots of natural ways to heal yourself by adjusting your diet slightly. Take some time and do a bit of research about your health. Instead of always looking for a pill to solve your health issues, look at alternative ways of eating to keep healthy.

In short, the best way to maintain a healthy body is to drink plenty of water, eat lots of fresh fruits and vegetables, and choose lean meats and fish, soy products, unsalted nuts, and beans and or/legumes as sources of protein . Get plenty of fiber from fruits, vegetables, and whole grain foods that are rich in nutrients, and avoid eating highly processed foods, bad fats, sugar, white flour, alcohol, and caffeine products. Try to limit the amount of pesticides, chemicals, and artificial sweeteners and flavors that you allow to go into your body. Think about what is in the food that you put into your body, and remember that the purpose of eating is to nourish your body.

CHAPTER 7

—*Problem Foods and Harmful Substances*—

Every item that enters your body has an impact of some kind. It is time to take a closer look at some of the foods that really have a negative impact on our bodies. These foods slow down our digestive system, take nutrients away from us, and keep us unhealthy and fat. They also block us from reaching our goals. Unfortunately, in the fast food world we exist in today, these foods are everywhere, and it's easy to just eat what's there without much thought, but this endangers our health. We really need to think about all the garbage and chemicals that we are continuously putting into our bodies. To ignore the negative effects of these foods is nothing short of ridiculous. If you want to stay healthy, listen up!

My son came home from school one day and told me about a movie that he watched at high school. The movie was called *Super Size Me*. He was very excited about it and suggested that we should rent the movie and all watch it together as a family. So that is what we did. The movie is actually a documentary about one man who eats nothing but fast food for 30 days and how it affects his health.

It also showcased how many chemicals and preservatives are in fast food. I would have to say that this movie cured me of my desire to eat at fast food restaurants.

If you have seen this movie, I would recommend that you watch it again. If you haven't seen it, I would strongly recommend that you rent it or even buy it. I am so grateful that I had a chance to watch this movie, because it really made me start to think of the effect that unhealthy foods have on our bodies. In this movie, a perfectly healthy, thin man went to a doctor and had a check-up of all his vital organs prior to starting the program to have a clear picture of the health of his body. He then proceeded to eat only fast food for one month and had regular checkups as the weeks went by. It was absolutely startling to see how much his body was affected in a negative way by eating fast food in such a short amount of time.

Since this movie was released, many of the fast food restaurants have made changes to their menus to make them healthier. I thought this was a great movie. However, I was saddened to hear that the school board stopped showing the movie in the schools for fear of lawsuits from the multi-million-dollar fast food chains.

So why is fast food so bad for you? It is full of salt, fat, sugar, and highly processed, high-calorie foods that are low in nutritional value. I think it is important to remember that everything that goes into your body creates some kind of reaction inside of you. The foods that you eat can either affect you in a good way or a bad way—there is no in-between.

I think it is important to remember the reasons our bodies need to eat particular foods. Many of us forget that food is fuel for our body. It is not meant to be eaten for enjoyment, fulfillment, or to satisfy our emotional needs. Food is required to sustain our lives and nothing more. This does not mean that you shouldn't enjoy your meal, but I think it is important to adjust your mental attitude to reflect the fact that we eat to live and to sustain life; we do not live to eat and enjoy food. This is a very simple fact to understand, and it will help you change your mental focus and unhealthy relationship that you may have with food.

Of course, there are some foods that are worse than others, so before you panic and think you won't be able to eat anything, let's look at some of the worst culprits. It is very important to pay attention to the way you feel after you eat. You will start to notice that certain foods will give you energy, and other foods will make you feel lethargic, lazy, bloated, and full of gas. The trick is to notice and understand the signals that your body is sending so that you will be able to see for yourself which foods you should be avoiding and which foods make you feel good.

Keep in mind that we are all human, and we cannot always eat perfectly. If you have a particularly bad meal, let it go and make a better choice for the next meal. The goal is to try to eat the best that you can whenever you can, and with time, it will become a habit for you to choose the healthier foods without even thinking about it.

I have certain foods that I have relegated to my own personal black list. These are foods that I try to avoid whenever possible. When I do eat them, I try to limit them to the smallest amount possible, remembering that you are what you eat and that if I want to feel good, I will need to make the best choices possible. The goal is to not be a perfect eater, but a better one, so as you become aware of how certain foods affect you, let your awareness increase and know you have a large degree of control over your health and appearance.

Sugar

Centuries ago, sugar was a very rare thing. Even up to the start of the twentieth century, it was seen as a rare treat and not something that permeated every meal. Sugar is very bad for the pH levels in your blood. It is acidic to your body and does not give you any nutrition. When you hear people talk about empty calories, they are often referring to a food that has high sugar content and no nutritional value. I would have to say that sugar is probably the number one item on my black list of foods I try to avoid.

To completely eliminate sugar from your diet is almost impossible because it is added to almost everything, including tobacco, cough syrup, pops, juices, breads, baked goods, soups, candy, chocolate, ice cream, cereals, salad dressings, and many more items. There is nothing wrong with having something sweet. However, if you look at the nutritional value of sugar, you will see that it is actually an antinutrient: a food that causes your body to lose nutrient value from eating it, rather than giving you nutrition. Sugar is full of calories and gives you no nutrition. It should be avoided most of the time.

If you are like most people, you are probably addicted to your sugary treats. If you can't seem to give them up at first, then you can simply shift the source. For example, instead of a candy bar, you might have a nice cup of tea or glass of lemonade. You are still getting your sugar fix until you can adjust to a no-sugar type of eating pattern, but you are lowering the amount of your sugar intake. It's kind of like a smoker who decreases their tobacco intake until they are weaned off the addiction.

I have found that agave nectar is a great alternative as a sweetener for my tea or for lemonade. It is also great as an alternative to pancake syrup or for use in baking. Another great alternative is stevia. Both of these items can be found at your local health-food stores or grocery stores. I particularly like using agave nectar because it does not affect your blood sugar levels the way that sugar would. It is a natural product, it tastes great, and it satisfies my sweet tooth. If you would like to get more information about the effects of sugar on your body, I would highly recommend that you purchase the book *Sugar Blues*, written by William Dufty. You can purchase it on Amazon.com. His book really exposes some of the harmful effects of sugar on our bodies that we are just beginning to understand, as the population has only been exposed to high sugar levels over the last fifty years or so. You will be absolutely astonished at the negative effects of sugar on your body.

Other ways to reduce sugar from your diet are:

- **Instead of drinking pop, try fruit juice with club soda. Or squeeze fresh lemon juice and make your own lemonade sweetened with agave nectar or stevia.**

- **When baking, try using half the recommended amount of sugar in your recipes or use a healthy alternative sweetener.**

- **Watch food labels for sucrose. This is another way of saying sugar. If the first three ingredients in the food that you are buying are sugar, sucrose, or sucralose, I would recommend that you put that item back on the shelf.**

- **Eat fresh fruit, which is naturally sweet and gives you some good nutritional value.**

Salt

Salt is another one of those items that seems to be in just about everything these days. I never add salt to my food anymore. However, if you eat out or buy a lot of fast food, prepackaged foods, or canned foods, you will be getting a lot of extra salt. It is a good idea to pay attention to what you are eating by reading labels and avoiding foods that have lots of extra salt in them. Even if you just buy those same foods in a low-sodium form, that is a start. Salt is also called sodium, so watch for that on your labels. It is true we need salt to survive, but we actually need very small amounts for our bodies to function, and we have become accustomed to salt overload. Why is salt so bad for you? It makes you retain water; it is hard on your organs, such as your liver and kidneys, which have to filter out the excess, and it can contribute to high blood pressure. While salt itself doesn't cause you to have a stroke, high blood pressure will.

Ways in which you can avoid salt:

·   **Avoid prepackaged foods such as crackers, chips, nuts, soy sauce, dressings, and canned soups, which are high in salt or sodium. Many food manufacturers offer unsalted brands of their foods or reduced-sodium options. Take a look at the labels on the foods you eat to become aware of all the extra additives that come in your prepackaged foods. Chinese food is full of salt, but you can ask for no salt and no MSG when ordering Chinese food. Most fast food outlets add salt to their foods, so, again, try to avoid fast food restaurants whenever possible.**

·   **When cooking at home, find other ways of seasoning your food. I use fresh lemon juice, dill, garlic powder, onions, fresh parsley, green onions, fresh celery, or garlic. You can also use other spices with less salt such as Mrs. Dash, hot chilies, basil, curry, pepper, dill, oregano, and other spices that do not have salt. If you are cooking soups or sauces, use fresh vegetables to add flavor to your sauces, such as onions, garlic, celery, tomatoes, and carrots.**

- When reading your labels, you should also try to avoid MSG (monosodium glutamate) and artificial sweeteners, such as aspartame. Many people have adverse reactions to these additives, such as bloating and headaches.

- Know what you are drinking. A big source of salt that most people don't even recognize is pop or soft drinks. Because they are usually sweet, we don't think of them as having loads of salt, but they do. And if you think that choosing the diet version is better, think again. Many diet soft drinks actually contain more salt than the regular version, and when you couple that with the artificial sweeteners in most diet drinks, it is a double whammy to your system.

Dairy Products

I personally do not eat any dairy products, as I have a severe intolerance to them. However, even if I did not have an intolerance to them, I would still want to avoid them. Dairy products are full of fat and bacteria, and often, added sugar and calories. Animal fats contained in dairy products are not good for you. These fats will clog your arteries, which increases your risk of high blood pressure and heart attacks or stroke, not to mention keeping you fat. It is also important to understand that most milk produced comes from cows that are injected with all sorts of growth hormones and bovine antibiotics. These flow through to the milk fat and can accumulate in your cells. None of these substances are natural to the human body, and over time, toxins build up and affect your health.

Dairy products are also bad for your body's pH levels, as they make your blood very acidic. If you choose to continue to eat dairy products, try to reduce the amount you eat and choose ones that are lower in fat and do not have added sugar or sweeteners in them. Many people are lactose intolerant or have adverse reactions when they eat dairy products. Some of those reactions are bloating, nasal congestion, arthritic joint pain, constipation, or diarrhea. Whenever your body is too acidic, your health is going to deteriorate, and dairy products are a big culprit.

Alcohol

Alcohol is another substance that is very acidic to our bodies, so you want to limit your consumption of it. It is particularly hard on your liver and kidneys, and beverages such as beer and wine contain many calories that do not give you any nutrition. The pop and mixers that go with the alcohol are full of added sugars and more calories. If you are a beer drinker, you are ingesting a great deal of yeast in your brew, which can cause you to feel bloated and gain weight.

In addition to calories, many wines are full of sulfites, which can cause migraines. If you are going to drink wine, choose an organic wine or a wine that is sulfite-free. Red wine can be beneficial in lowering blood cholesterol. However, you want to limit your intake to one glass per day and avoid the wines with sulfites and other additives that are harmful to your body.

Alcohol can lead to addiction if you use it as a coping mechanism or if you drink too much and too often. In large amounts, alcohol can cause cirrhosis of your liver. Like most items on my black list, alcohol has no nutritional value, is acidic to your body, causes dehydration, and is full of empty calories.

Bad Fats

Your body needs a variety of fats to be healthy, but you want to make sure that you get the right kind of fats and avoid the harmful ones. Again, the body's chemistry is a balance, and while it needs things like fat, that doesn't mean that more is better. I try to avoid hard animal fats, which are found in red meats, cheese, high-fat dairy products; lard, which is used in many pastries; and hydrogenated fats, which are found in many fast food items and margarines.

Sometimes, it is difficult to get enough of the right kind of healthy fats in your diet, like the omegas that come from fish oil or nuts. I try to take an omega 3-6-9 tablet each day that has the good fats that our bodies need. I use cold-pressed olive oil in my salads with a little lemon juice and garlic or other seasonings and fresh herbs. Salmon and most fish are a good source of healthy fat.

White Flour

We know that flour comes from grain. But have you ever seen white grain? I haven't, and if there is no white grain, how in the world can there be white flour? The truth is that white flour has been processed so much that by the time you eat it, there is very little nutrition or fiber left in it. Mills work to make the flour so fine and fluffy that the grain is annihilated—then they bleach it. Yes, with actual bleach! Otherwise it would never be white. In our quest for pretty food, we often end up with worthless food, from a nutritional standpoint.

I try not to eat too much bread or grains, but when I do eat them, I gravitate toward the high fiber, multi-grain choices. The problem with white processed flour is that it is everywhere, and we eat much more of it than we realize. White flour is found in battered fish, donuts, pastries, cookies, and bread. These products are also full of salt, sugar, and unhealthy fats, so the flour is compounding the effect of empty calories.

Pesticides, Hormones, and Other Harmful Substances in Our Food.

It may seem way off-topic to talk about pesticides and chemicals on a black list of foods, but we eat them all the time without even knowing it. We are told repeatedly how good it is to eat lots of fresh fruits and vegetables. Knowing what I know now, I am surprised that there are no warning labels on our fresh fruits and vegetables that inform us of all the chemicals that are sprayed all over them. This is done in an industry effort to ward off pests that might make the fruit look ugly—and thus not sell as well as the pretty fruit. Some fruits and vegetables are worse than others.

I started noticing that whenever I would stop by the local fruit stand and buy cherries or nectarines, my mouth would get swollen and I would get a rash on my lips and mouth after eating what I had bought. This was not a reaction to the fruit, but a reaction to the chemicals sprayed all over the fruit. I guess the insects are smarter than we are, as they know better than to eat this perfect-looking fruit. We still need the nutritional value from fruits and vegetables in our diet. So what can you do?

You should buy organic fruits and vegetables whenever possible. I know that organic vegetables cost more, but the prices have come down substantially in the past few years, and as more consumers use organic foods, the price will continue to decrease. You should also wash your fruits and vegetables well before you eat them. Most of the chemicals are on the skin of the fruit or vegetable, so if you peel them, you will remove most of the chemicals. Some of the more delicate fruits like grapes, cherries, nectarines, and peaches have more chemicals on the portion of the food that you will eat, so it is a good idea to spray those foods with a vegetable wash to make sure that you get most of the chemicals off before you eat them. Broccoli should also be cleaned well. I personally try to buy organic broccoli whenever I can, as it can be hard to get this type of produce really clean.

SUZANNE
PANTAZIS

Over the last few years, there have been many issues with chemicals or dangerous substances that have gotten into our food supply. Not long ago, there was a large recall of spinach because it was contaminated with dangerous salmonella bacteria. A decade ago, a genetically engineered corn called StarLink corn was grown by numerous farmers in the United States in anticipation of approval by the FDA. They were surprised when the government deemed it too dangerous due to adverse allergic reactions it caused in some people. Still, some of this corn entered the food supply, and many people were made ill. To this day there are still traces of StarLink corn in many of the corn products we eat.

One of the areas that people don't necessarily consider when thinking of chemicals in our food is the smoked meats we often eat. Smoke contains chemicals that are carcinogenic—meaning they have been shown to cause cancer. They also are often infused with a great deal of salt and preservatives that the body does not handle well.

Speaking of meat, do you know what the chicken or cow you are eating was fed before it landed on your dinner table? Many of our fish and meats come from animals that are pumped full of steroids, hormones, and antibiotics. When you eat those animals, you also are ingesting those substances into your body. Are the substances used to fatten up animals also fattening you up? Did you know that farmed salmon are up to ten times higher in pesticides like PCBs compared to wild salmon? This is just another way that we end up taking substances into our bodies that may be harmful to us. If you can choose hormone-free or wild fish or meat, I think these are wise choices.

You may think that the body eliminates these pesticides and chemicals, but you would be wrong. Chemicals, toxins, and heavy metals build up in our bodies over our entire lives, so the effect is cumulative.

Fast Food and Highly Processed Food

The difference between fast food and highly processed food can cause some confusion, so we'll clear that up first. Fast food is generally served by fast food restaurants whose menus contain a lot of fried foods (like French fries), as well as high-calorie foods (like shakes and ice cream creations). They tend to have high-calorie sauces or dips (like for chicken nuggets) and serve many of their items on a white bun with a large soft drink. These foods are full of fat, salt, white flour, and empty calories. In addition, some items are full of artificial sweeteners, preservatives, and other chemicals. When you tell someone that fast food is bad for them, they will agree, but they often don't understand how bad it is. The typical fast food meal of a burger, fries, and a large soft drink can easily have more than 1,500 calories—almost the entire daily intake amount for most people. Not to mention the fat and salt, which are often far in excess of our entire daily needs. When you add to this the fact that this meal is almost bereft of any nutritional value, it becomes clear why many obese people are also on the edge of being malnourished. Their bodies are getting an overload of calories but very little of the nutrients they need.

Highly processed packaged foods are things like heat-and-eat meals from the freezer, prepackaged crackers, cookies, cakes, Toaster Pastries, donuts, pop, energy drinks, pastries, canned pasta dishes, many canned soups, potato chips, sugary low fiber cereals, candies, and ice cream, to name just a few. They are quick and easy to eat, but offer little in the way of nutrition and are highly acidic foods for pH levels in your body.

I remember running into a colleague of mine at the local supermarket one day. I noticed that he was buying about 30 packages of little toaster pastries. He was thin, didn't smoke, exercised, and seemed like a pretty healthy fellow. I was shocked that he would be purchasing so much garbage food. I remember commenting on how bad that stuff was for him. He laughed and said he didn't care because they tasted good. Oddly enough, he died six months later of cancer at the young age of forty-nine. The cancer started in his digestive system. After he was diagnosed with cancer, he made radical changes to his diet to try to eat in a more healthy way. He told me how he had lived on a diet of Pop-Tarts, pop, candies, and chips and how he rarely ate fruits and vegetables. By the time he realized how harmful his eating habits were to his health, it was too late for him. The cancer had moved into his bones. I have no doubt in my mind that if he had changed his eating habits ten years earlier, he would still be alive today.

Prescription Drugs

Prescription and over-the-counter medications can compromise your digestive system, and they can also cause many side effects. I will tell you right now that I am not a fan of the pharmaceutical industry. They make billions of dollars each year treating your symptoms. If you suddenly heal yourself, they are going to lose money. They have a vested interest in keeping you sick. I prefer to try to fix the root cause of any illness in my body, rather than continually take medications to treat the symptoms but not the root cause. I have become a big advocate of naturopathic medicine, which tends to look for the root cause of illness, rather than treating the symptoms with synthetic chemicals that can cause harmful side effects. There is a lot of information available these days on the Internet and in your local library. If you are sick, take some time to do a bit of research, and don't just take the standard answers from medical professionals. Get a second opinion, and listen to the signals your body is giving you.

Let me give you an example of my experience with prescription drugs. I was in a bad car accident, and I was having some muscle aches and pain. When this accident happened, I had already lost a lot of weight, my blood pressure was normal, and I was eating well and exercising regularly. Overall, I was pretty healthy. After the accident, I was given a pain medication that made me terribly drowsy, sick to my stomach, and constipated. When I complained, my doctor put me on another medication that caused my menstrual cycles to get all out of whack, and I was bleeding all of the time. I also could feel a strange sensation in my chest, so I decided to discontinue that medication. This medication was later recalled from the market because it was found to cause serious heart damage. The doctor then switched me to another medication that seemed to help with few side effects, or so I thought.

A little while later, I went to the doctor, and when she checked my blood pressure, it was high. I was surprised by this because I was doing everything right as far as my eating, exercising, drinking water, resting, avoiding salt, sugar, coffee, and alcohol, and I was slowly losing weight. She said that I needed to really watch my salt intake and fats, and she would check my blood pressure again on the next visit. I followed her instructions and went back to see her again, and she was still very concerned with my high blood pressure. She told me if I couldn't get my blood pressure down within two weeks, she would have to start me on blood pressure medication. There are many negative side effects from many blood pressure medications, including irreversible kidney damage.

I was puzzled and stunned by this sudden rise in my blood pressure. It did not make sense to me. I decided that I would go on the Internet and look up information about the medication that I was taking for my muscle aches and pain. Not surprisingly, I found that this particular medication had a side effect of causing high blood pressure. I called my doctor and mentioned this to her, and she suggested that I stop taking the medication to see what would happen. I stopped the medication and went back to see her two weeks later. When she checked my blood pressure, it was perfectly normal. I wondered to myself what would have happened to me if I hadn't look into this on my own. I would probably be taking

SUZANNE
PANTAZIS

the same medication, plus the blood pressure medication, and who knows what sort of health problems I would have created for myself by taking those drugs. I was surprised that my doctor would not have thought about the link with the medication, but like most doctors, they can only remember so much information, and they don't necessarily link a particular symptom to a drug they prescribed. From that day on, I decided to pay more attention to what I allow to go into my body. I have spoken to so many people who have had similar stories of illnesses being caused or worsened by prescription drugs. So please take the time to research what you are putting into your body before you blindly follow your doctor's orders. If you are not well, consider seeing a naturopathic doctor for another point of view.

Taking Baby Steps to Eating Healthier

I know that fast food is easy, but understand that it is a trade-off. Are you willing to perhaps trade a shorter life span for a few minutes today? Eating healthy can also be easy if you plan in advance. If you want something fast and easy, here are a few suggestions:

- **Prewashed organic salad mixes are a great way to quickly get some fresh vegetables into your diet.**

- **If you need to grab something quick, fresh fruit, unsalted nuts, and seeds are foods that are nutritious and easy to grab when you are on the run.**

- **Frozen vegetables, frozen fruits, and/or fish fillets are good foods to have on hand in your freezer that can be quickly reheated and made into a healthy meal.**

- **You can eat leftovers from the night before or have lean oven-roasted lunch meats. (I avoid the smoked meats, which are full of salt and other chemicals that have been directly linked to cancer.)**

- **If you have a little time on the weekend or at night, you can chop fresh fruits and veggies and cook larger quantities of healthy foods and snacks that will last all week.**

- **I will often boil some eggs at the start of the week and have them in the fridge so that I can quickly get some protein. They are great mashed with a little mayonnaise and green onion.**

If you can, plan ahead to try and keep healthy foods at home so that you can quickly make a healthy meal. This way, you will not need to eat out at fast food restaurants or eat highly processed foods. It may take a little more time, but it is worth it in the long run. It is also more expensive to eat out, so try to make the effort to plan ahead to eat healthy and save money. When you cook at home, you know what is going into your meals. You can cut back on the salt and fat and fill your meals with good, wholesome, nutritious food that is full of quality ingredients and free from additives and chemicals that you don't want or need.

If you are going to cook at any time of the week, you may as well cook a larger amount so that you can have leftovers or can freeze extra portions for the days when you don't have as much time. I usually don't work on Saturday and Sunday, so I will shop on Saturday and plan my meals for the week. On Sundays, I will try and make a nice dinner with leftovers to carry me through for lunch or supper on Monday. For example, I might roast a chicken with potatoes and carrots and onions. For Monday, I can have some leftovers with a salad for dinner. If I need a quick shot of protein, I may have a small piece of chicken with a piece of fruit as I run out the door on Monday to work.

Soups and chilies are also good items that you can make and put away portions for other meals on another day. I always make sure that I have lots of fresh or frozen fruit in the house for a quick, nutritious snack. Other good items to have on hand are unsalted nuts, seeds, canned tuna, eggs, lean lunch meats, ready-to-eat salad mixes, tomatoes, carrots, cucumbers, and red peppers. This way, you can nibble on some vegetables or make a small salad very quickly. Even if you are not much of a cook, you can still eat healthier by cooking frozen vegetables or prepared frozen healthy meals, such as Lean Cuisine or Healthy Choice meals. These are better than a greasy burger and fries and have more nutrition.

It is also so important to have a nice supply of water to drink. If you don't like tap water, invest in a water cooler and buy the large bottles of water that you can use to always have nice water to drink. I personally don't like the tap water, so I always make sure I have bottled water or herbal teas I can drink to make sure that I get the fluids that my body needs to function properly.

As consumers start to demand healthier foods, the retailers and fast food outlets will start to supply healthier options. Since the making of the movie *Super Size Me*, you will notice that many fast food outlets now offer salads, fresh fruits, lean meats, and healthier foods. You can find many healthier premade meals in your grocery stores these days, too. Health-food stores have many healthy choices. You just have to make a change to your pattern of eating. If you are not happy with the choices at your local supermarket, give them your opinion and let them know what you would like to see as a consumer. Your opinion and your voice matter.

Keep Learning

It is impossible to eat perfectly all the time and avoid all the problem foods and chemicals that we are constantly exposed to. However, if you can try to limit your intake, I know that you will lower your risk of developing cancer, and you will be healthier.

Eating isn't about perfection; it's about making those small changes that can substantially add to how you feel and extend your life span.

Your body has the ability to filter out many of the harmful foods and chemicals that you eat but not all, and the more chemicals that go into your body, the harder your liver, kidneys, and other vital organs have to work. When your liver and kidneys get overworked, they will deteriorate and not function properly or simply shut down completely. When this happens, your body can become very toxic, and you will get very sick and eventually die.

You have it within your power to change small habits that you engage in every day that will have a long-term impact on your health. You also have the ability to choose to feel better and look better. These changes are immeasurable but contribute significantly to your overall happiness and joy. Only by continually educating yourself will you really understand how to work with your body and be the best possible version of yourself. Feeling good and looking good sound simple, but they require thought and knowledge. You are worth that knowledge. You deserve to have a happy, healthy life. Choose now to start taking those small steps that will get you there.

CHAPTER 8

—Exercise—

I am sure that you have been told many times before that exercise is important for your health. I heard it many times as well but never did anything about it. I really discounted the benefits of exercise and rationalized that I was too busy to exercise. I did not want to go to a gym to publicly display how out of shape I was. No thanks!

As a parent, I always made sure that my children were involved in sports to keep them healthy and active. I would take them to their soccer games, karate classes, swimming lessons, skiing lessons, and a whole variety of other activities. However, I never took the time to exercise myself. I always thought that I did not have the time to fit exercise into my life, and I was always too tired to exercise, anyway.

When you are young, you don't think twice about age or how food and exercise affect your body, but this oversight can really trick you into believing you don't need exercise. You do need it, and for many reasons. The benefits of exercise are multilayered and begin with the fact that exercise keeps your muscles toned and your body strong. The old saying, "Use it or lose it" is true. The more you use your muscles, the stronger and more defined they become. This makes you stronger, and it improves your appearance. If you don't exercise, your muscles tend to atrophy, which produces saggy, ill-defined areas of the body. Without that muscle tone, you will also experience pain and weakness, as the muscles are designed to hold your bones in proper alignment. If you don't exercise, those bones tend to twist and turn in unnatural ways, causing stress and strain in your joints and back.

When you exercise, you are also burning calories, which will help you to lose weight or even to maintain a good body weight. When you exercise, your heart rate elevates and stays elevated even after your exercise is finished. This improves your endurance and builds muscle, which burns more fat. So if you are physically fit, then even standing still you will naturally burn more calories than someone who doesn't exercise. This speeds up your metabolism.

When you exercise, you also allow the body to sweat, which is another way it gets rid of toxins and impurities. While it isn't necessary to sweat a lot to get a good workout, it helps the body function better overall.

For years, I had an extremely negative mindset about exercise, and I'm sure there are many other people who currently feel the same way. I think it is important to try to change your mind set about exercise if you have a negative opinion about it. You will also want to keep things interesting for yourself. Exercise should be fun and relaxing for you. You don't want to view it as a chore or something that you dislike to do. When I first started exercising, I hated it! I did view it as a chore, and I did not look forward to it at all. The reason for this is because I would try to exercise like a fit 20-year-old, and I was actually an out-of-shape 35-year-old with a bad back and a bad attitude. I would overdo things and hurt so badly for days afterward that it really discouraged me from wanting to exercise. I could not imagine how anyone could possibly enjoy it.

It is important not to go from one extreme to the other. That is what I did in the past. I would go months without exercise and then get myself all worked up and excited about getting into shape. I might impulsively join a gym, buy a workout video, or purchase the latest exercise gadget advertised on television. I would be full of vim and vigor and exercise like a maniac. Typically, I would end up pulling a muscle, wearing myself out, or realizing that I had no chance of keeping up with the Tae Bo video or the latest aerobics video. I got discouraged. I also felt a lot of pain from overdoing it, and this added to my negative view on exercise. In hindsight, what I really should have done was gradually increase my level of activity while decreasing the amount of time I spent in front of a television set or computer screen.

I realized that I needed to take things slower and make exercise a permanent habit in my life instead of an all-or-nothing proposition every few months. When I first decided to make a conscious effort to start exercising, I would just go for a short walk every night after dinner. It was a little bit of time that I would take for myself to do something good for me. I also thought that if I took time to be healthier, I would be better able to look after my family and to enjoy life with them. At the rate I was going on the unhealthy path I was on, I knew my body would start to deteriorate, and that would mean less time to be with my family. So I started my evening walks around my neighborhood. My children were still fairly young, so I stayed close to home, which meant walking around my block repeatedly. I would keep my cell phone with me so that if anything happened while I was out walking, they could call to reach me and I could call to reach them.

Once I got out there and started exercising, I realized that I really enjoyed it. It was a break for me. It gave me a chance to clear my thoughts and quietly reflect on things. It helped to reduce my stress levels after a busy day, and it also helped me to digest my food after eating. I had suffered with arthritic pain for many years and noticed that my arthritis seemed to improve with the walking and moving around. I didn't know it at the time, but keeping active and getting your joints moving helps to relieve stiff muscle aches and pains. It also increases the blood flow in your body, which helps it work more efficiently at every task, including improving digestion. Exercise is a wonderful way to relieve stress. When you exercise, your body releases endorphins, which make you feel good and improve your mood.

Endorphins are chemicals the body produces known as neurotransmitters, which function to transmit electrical signals within the nervous system. Endorphins interact with the opiate receptors in the brain to reduce our perception of pain and act similarly to drugs, such as morphine and codeine. In contrast to the opiate drugs, however, activation of the opiate receptors by the body's endorphins does not lead to addiction or dependence. In addition to decreased pain, secretion of endorphins leads to feelings of euphoria, a decrease in appetite, the release of sex hormones, and an enhancement of the immune response.

Endorphin levels attained through exercise varies among individuals. This means that two people who exercise at the same level will not necessarily produce similar levels of endorphins. Even if you don't participate in strenuous athletics, moderate exercise will still increase your body's endorphin levels.

In addition to simply feeling better through the release of chemicals such as endorphins, exercising on a regular basis can reduce your blood pressure, lower your weight, and help your metabolism by increasing muscle mass. More muscle mass makes you stronger and tones your body, and since muscle burns more calories than fat, having more muscle means your body uses more calories, even at a standstill.

Exercise is also a great way to socialize and meet new people. No matter what type of exercise you decide to do, it is a positive way to get out and meet people or to spend time with the people that you already know. One of the best benefits is that you are meeting like-minded people who also want to stay healthy and improve their appearance, and this is encouraging. I have met lots of people at my gym. We encourage each other and also help each other out by pushing each other beyond our comfort zones or with suggestions on different ways to work out. I have developed friendships that completely revolve around exercise, rather than those that just revolve around eating or sedentary activities. It is nice to have friends who enjoy getting out and doing something physical.

Exercise can be fun. It doesn't have to be hard. There are so many fun ways to get some exercise. It doesn't have to be a boring, painful workout all by yourself on a treadmill. A few suggestions for some fun activities that you can do on your own—or with a friend who can make exercising lots of fun—might be to play tennis, soccer, basketball, baseball, racquetball, or any other competitive sports. You might go to the local beach or swimming pool. When the weather is warm, there is nothing better than a nice hike in the outdoors to someplace beautiful and scenic. Some people prefer to play a round of golf or go for a bike ride or a mountain bike ride. You are limited only by your imagination to find fun ways to keep yourself active and fit. As you start to develop ways to get out there and get moving, you will find that you will look forward to exercise, rather than dreading it.

Another way to get yourself moving is to tackle some chores around the house. This is a great way to get moving and also to feel good about your surroundings. You would be surprised how many calories you can burn by vacuuming, dusting, washing floors, taking out the garbage, cleaning bathrooms, or cleaning out the garage. Do that yard work that you've been putting off, such as weeding the flower bed, raking leaves, mowing the lawn, or even shoveling snow in the winter. Keeping busy and active is a great step toward being less sedentary. So if you really need to get your car washed, get busy and wash that car. You don't have to do jumping jacks and sit-ups to get some exercise in. Just get moving!

If you want to make a permanent change, it is always a good idea to substitute a bad habit with a good one. If you normally turn on the television set when you get home from work or when you first get up in the morning, change your habit. Get yourself off that couch. Turn on your music instead of the television or computer. Tell yourself that you are not going to turn on the television set for at least three hours after getting home or after getting up in the morning. You will be amazed at how much extra time you will have on your hands and how many things you will accomplish.

Now, I already said that, at first, I wasn't really thrilled about the idea of exercise, so I used nearly every excuse in the book to avoid it. See if some of these sound familiar:

Excuse: I don't have time to exercise.

Reality Check: Saying that you don't have time to exercise is like saying that you don't have time to eat or breathe. Your body needs to exercise. You just have not made exercise a priority in your life. If you own a television set or a home computer, simply turning them off for one hour each day will provide time to exercise. If you go to the bar for a drink after work, skipping this activity a couple of times per week—or even eliminating it completely—will give you your time to exercise. Replace your bad habits with good ones, and you will find that you really do have time to exercise. You just need to make exercise more of a priority in your life.

Excuse: I can't afford the money to join a gym or take fitness classes.

Reality Check: You don't need to join a gym or take fitness classes. Implementing exercise into your life doesn't have to cost you anything. It does not cost you anything to go for a walk or to dance to music at home. There are lots of fun ways to exercise at little or no cost to you. Sometimes you will need to purchase a piece of sports equipment to help you with exercise, but that can be as inexpensive as buying a basketball, a tennis racket, a good pair of running shoes, a bathing suit, or shorts. Go shoot baskets at your local park or high school. If you can't afford new equipment, buy second-hand. Don't let money be your excuse. If you can't afford to exercise, you really need to look at what your money-spending priorities are. How much do you spend each month on Cablevision, Internet, cell phones, eating out, and buying junk food, or on prescriptions or over-the-counter medications to correct issues caused by additional weight? You choose what to spend your money on, so spend it on exercise, not junk.

Excuse: I have a medical condition that prevents me from exercising.

Reality Check: There are lots of ways to exercise, even if you have a medical condition. Many medical conditions are helped by exercise, especially arthritis-type conditions, because the movement of the joints helps to loosen things up, and this helps to relieve pain. You will, of course, want to talk with your doctor to determine different ways in which you can increase your level of activity. You may have to start things off slowly, but I am sure there is some type of activity that you can do, despite your medical condition. We all get injured or sick from time to time, and this may force us to stop exercising while we are healing, but don't let that be an excuse to completely become sedentary.

Excuse: My friend and I were supposed to go to the gym together, but she cancelled on me.

Reality Check: This is a common excuse, but it is a lame excuse at best. You are the one who is in control of your body. If you plan to exercise, and your exercise partner doesn't make it, then go on without them. You may have to do another form of exercise, but if you are ready to go and work out, just do it! It is a good idea to have a set date and time when you want to exercise. You can invite a friend to join you, but in the event that the friend doesn't show, you need to be strong and go on your own. Take responsibility for you and your future.

Excuse: I have small children and I don't have a babysitter, so it is hard for me to exercise.

Reality Check: I know that it is hard to fit exercise in, especially when you have small children, but there is always a way if you really want to make things work. Here are a few suggestions: Walk with your children to a park and play games with them. Push them on the swing, lift them up and down on the slide or the teeter-totter, play tag with them, or simply keep active by letting them run loose while you chase after them. Take your child to a local swimming pool and swim around with them. You will find that if you exercise with your children, they will be healthier, and they will sleep better for you after using up all that childhood energy exercising.

You can also plan your exercise while your child is napping without leaving home at all. When your child goes down for a nap, do some push-ups, walk on a treadmill, or get on an exercise bike while they sleep. Put on your iPod or music and dance your calories away. If you have a close friend or family member who also has a small child, you can trade babysitting time. You can look after their child while they do errands or chores, and then they can look after your child while you exercise.

Excuse: I planned to exercise, but something always comes up that prevents me from going to do my exercise.

Reality Check: Make an unbreakable appointment for exercise. If something else comes up, the appointment is set. It is no different than if you had a doctor's appointment scheduled and someone asked you to do something for them or with them at that time. You would tell them that you can't see them or help them because you have an appointment. This is an appointment that is just as important as the doctor's appointment—even more important, in fact. Having said that, you want to carefully think about the time of day that you want to do your exercise so that you won't have things come up that will throw you out of your routine. I try to get up earlier in the morning and exercise before I go to work. I find that very little will come up in the early morning hours that will prevent me from exercising. However, you have to find the time that works for you.

Excuse: I am too out of shape to exercise. It is embarrassing to go out in public and exercise. People will laugh at me.

Reality Check: The reason why you are out of shape is because you don't exercise. If you are embarrassed about your appearance, you can start to exercise at home. You can simply start out by going for walks or by doing chores around your house or in your yard. I remember how awkward I felt when I first joined my gym. I wasn't sure how to use the equipment, and I was really out of shape. What I found was that people actually admired me for making the effort to get out there and do something about my poor physical condition. They were very helpful in showing me how to use the equipment and really encouraged me to keep on working out. I watched other people use the equipment, and I read books about proper ways to use the equipment. Before long, I was just another member at the gym who was getting into great shape. So try to be brave and just get started.

Excuse: I get plenty of exercise at work. I don't need to exercise after a hard day's work.

Reality Check: You know what? You might be right on this one. If you are doing a very physical job, then you may be getting enough exercise during the day. However, most people do not do nearly the exercise they think they do at work. I would still recommend taking an hour a day for yourself in which you exercise your mind and nurture your spirit. Turn off the TV or computer for one hour a day and spend that time doing something good for yourself. This time could be used to meditate and reduce your stress. You could use this time to focus on goals or business ideas that could help you to be more successful in your life. You could do yoga or stretching exercises to help to relieve tension in your muscles. You could go to the swimming pool and relax in the hot tub. Take some time for yourself in a productive way. Take this time to look within and see what improvements you would like to make in your life to make yourself happier and healthier.

Baby Steps, Baby Steps

If you don't have a regular exercise routine, it is sometimes hard to get started. So let me give you a few pointers to help set yourself up for success. Before you get started, you need to take an honest look at your current level of health and fitness. No matter what condition you are in, there is some way that you can exercise. As in any lifestyle change, you do not want to do things too drastically, or you will likely injure yourself or get discouraged when you wake up aching all over from doing too much, too quickly. With all the changes that I am suggesting in this book, it is important to try to slowly implement permanent changes that you can sustain on a permanent basis.

For most people, when it comes to changing their lifestyle, they come up against the old struggle of time versus money. You may find that you have the money to join a gym, take exercise classes, and be involved in a number of other healthy activities—but you don't have the time. You are so busy making that money that there seems to be little room left for something like exercise. On the other hand, you may have all the time in the world, but find that you don't have the funds to join a gym or take classes.

If you have money, but you don't seem to have enough time, try to find ways to use your money to buy you some time. You can hire a housekeeper to save you some time cleaning your house . Use this time to exercise and look after yourself. Perhaps you can hire an assistant to assist you to free up some time. When I am very busy, I will just eat more often at restaurants where I can get a healthy meal to free up my time from shopping, cooking and cleaning up. If you keep working too hard and don't take time to take care of yourself, you will eventually make yourself sick and then you won't be able to work at all.

What I am proposing is small, incremental steps to get you started on the path to change. If you are constantly working and busy, then look for little incremental ways to introduce exercise into what you already do. If you work in an office building, take the stairs. When you run errands, park in a distant parking spot and walk. Put a small set of dumbbells in your desk drawer and lift weights while you talk on the phone with customers. All of these are small incremental ideas that, when combined with healthier eating habits and drinking more water, will make a big difference in your overall health.

If you have time on your hands, then look for things you can do around the house for exercise. I knew an older lady who used canned vegetables as weights, and she exercised to keep her arthritis in check. You can also volunteer to work with children or coach a sports team—anything that will get you out and moving. You don't have to join a gym or any other regimented exercise program. By simply making little changes in what you do, you can introduce motion and calorie-burning activities into your life, and that is the whole point.

If you are going to be effective at implementing exercise into your life, it is very important to plan things in advance. The first thing that you should try to do is to figure out the right time for you to exercise. You want to choose a time of day when you will have good energy levels and little chance of something else coming up that could result in your having to cancel your exercise plans. I vary the times and the ways in which I exercise during the year. I live in a four-season climate in British Columbia. In the summer, I like to get outside to do my exercise. The days are much longer, so I can exercise very early in the morning until very late at night. However, in the winter months, the hours of daylight are reduced, so I need to move indoors to get my exercise done. On my days off, I have much more flexibility, so that leaves me open to many more options. I try to exercise in some way five to six days a week. I try to make it a point to take one day off to let my body rest and recuperate.

If you are just starting to exercise, I would try to exercise three times per week and gradually increase that amount when you feel ready. I usually exercise for one hour each day, but I may take longer to exercise if I am doing a fun activity like golfing, skiing, or bike riding. I find that for me personally, it is easier to get my exercise done first thing in the morning. This way, it's done at the beginning of the day and actually puts me in a really good and energetic mood for the rest of the day. It is important to make sure that I get to sleep earlier to accommodate getting up earlier. Depending on your lifestyle, you may need to exercise during a lunch break, after work, or after dinner. Take a good look at your current schedule and try to find the right time to fit exercise into your life. Whatever time that you decide to exercise, make a firm appointment with yourself to exercise during the time that you have chosen on the days that you have chosen.

Once you have chosen a time that works for you, you need to choose the type of activity that you would like to do. Try to mix things up so you don't get bored with the same routine. It is also important to try to exercise many different muscles in your body, and then give them time to rest and heal in between exercise sessions. You don't want to just do one type of exercise. When I go to the gym, I do cardio exercise every other day, and I do weight training on the days in between cardio days. I try to work the muscles in my upper body one day, stomach muscles and low back muscles on another day, and lower body muscles the third day. This allows the different muscle groups to relax in between sessions so that I don't strain or overwork one particular muscle group. If you overdo it one day and injure yourself, make sure that you give that muscle time to heal before resuming your regular exercise of that particular muscle group or modify your routine so that you avoid using the muscle that is injured.

If you decide to join a gym and do weight training exercises, take some time to educate yourself on the proper way to do the exercises. There are plenty of books out there on weight training and exercise, and most gyms offer some free education from an onsite trainer. These are all great tools to help you get started. You may also want to consider working with a personal trainer at first to make sure that you are using the equipment properly so that you don't injure yourself and get the most benefit out of your exercise routine.

A BETTER
LIFE AWAITS

Getting Back on Track

I find that once I get myself into a routine, then exercise just becomes a regular part of my life. I know that I exercise on certain days at certain times. However, sometimes unexpected events happen in your life that gets you out of your routine. I find that the most common thing that gets me out of my routine is an injury, an illness, or a holiday. Over the summer, I was out hiking and badly twisted my ankle. I was told to keep off of my ankle for the next two to four weeks. I knew that if I did not rest my ankle it would not heal well, so I followed my doctor's orders and I did not exercise for about two weeks. This messed up my routine. I was so used to exercising, and now suddenly I couldn't exercise.

I decided to use this time to spend more time doing meditation, and I made it my deliberate intention that I would get back into my exercise routine on a certain date. It was hard to get back into my routine after this injury. I normally exercise in the morning before I go to work, so I had gotten kind of used to sleeping in later and taking it easy for a while. I also noticed that I had gained about five pounds during this break in my routine, my pants felt a little tighter, and my energy level was quite a bit lower. Also, because I had injured my ankle, I could not exercise at the level of intensity that I was used to. I had to ease myself back into exercise. The worst thing you can do is to overdo things and get injured again, so I wanted to ease myself back into exercising slowly.

When I started back, I did cut myself a bit of slack. I did not want to get discouraged, so I started by doing a lighter workout than normal. The most important thing to me was to get used to getting up earlier and making it a habit to do my exercise each morning. I knew that once I started to get back into my routine, I would slowly be able to increase my intensity as my body got stronger and my energy levels started to return back to normal.

I find that the hardest part of exercising is just getting started or getting to the gym or place where you plan to do your exercise. I know that if I can just get myself to the gym, or get myself out of bed and onto the treadmill, half the battle has been won by just showing up. There are going to be days when your energy levels are higher or lower. As long as you commit to exercising at a certain time on a certain date, you will start to see some results. If you normally walk for two miles but one day are feeling really tired and lethargic, just slow things down a little. Remember to listen to your body. You don't want to let yourself get run down or discouraged. If you push too hard, too often, you will end up making yourself sick or injuring yourself. So don't be overly hard on yourself when you are first starting to exercise. No one ran a marathon the first day! Just get to the gym or to the exercise class or to the place where you are planning to exercise.

I can't say that I have ever gone to work out and regretted it later. I always feel good about myself after I finish my workout or my exercise routine, and I always make it a point to congratulate myself for a good workout. I will pat myself on the shoulder and say, "Good job, Suzanne! You were tired today, but you got out of bed and made it to the gym. You had a great workout! Way to go!"

Keep a positive attitude with regard to exercise, and you will reap the rewards of having a healthier, stronger, and better-looking body as a result of it.

CHAPTER 9

—Rest and Stress—

Life can be very busy at times, and we often don't take sufficient time to slow down to give our bodies, minds, and spirits sufficient time to rest and regenerate. The time we take to rest and regenerate is a crucial part of feeling good and being healthy.

I know that when I am tired and I don't have time to rest, I will tend to eat more than I would normally because I am trying to give myself energy. I find that when I am tired, I am more likely to snap at others or to make mistakes I would not normally make if I was not so tired. I will also be less productive at work than I would be if I was well-rested. It also makes it harder to keep on track with healthy eating when you are tired.

Stress and Your Adrenal Glands

If you suffer from chronic fatigue syndrome , fibromyalgia or if you have a very stressful life, you may be suffering from adrenal fatigue. Some estimates indicate that as many as 70%, or more, of individuals with Chronic Fatigue Syndrome or Fibromyalgia have an underlying adrenal condition. When you are under a lot of stress, your adrenal glands react by releasing various hormones to help you deal with the stress. It is a defence mechanism. Have you ever been in a highly stressful situation and felt the rush of adrenaline in your body? This is created by the proper functioning of your adrenal glands. If you have a particularly stressful event in your life, or if you are subjected to ongoing stress for long periods of time, your adrenal glands stop functioning properly, resulting in Adrenal Fatigue. Some of the symptoms of adrenal fatigue are: Fatigue, Insomnia, Salt and Sugar cravings, slow healing after an illness , osteoporosis, constant worrying, high blood pressure, disinterest in sex, aches and pains, arthritic pain, anxiety, difficulty getting up in the morning, insomnia at night, weight gain primarily in the stomache area.

How to recover from or prevent Adrenal Fatigue.

If you suspect that you may have adrenal fatigue there are saliva tests that can be done to measure your hormone levels to determine if you might have adrenal fatigue. If you are suffering from adrenal fatigue, you should avoid the use of stimulants or caffeine contained in coffee, energy drinks, alcohol , wake-up pills etc. You need to let your body get the rest that it needs. If you are tired, get some sleep. Try to reduce your stress in healthy ways. You also need to get the nutrition that your body needs by eating a diet that is full of nutritious foods like lots of fresh fruit & vegetables and whole grains, while reducing refined carbohydrates & fast food. If you don't deal with your adrenal fatigue, you may develop diabetes, autoimmune disorders, chronic fatigue, fibromyalgia and/or hypoglycaemia.

Getting the Rest You Need

In a perfect world, we would put our heads down on our pillows each night and have eight hours of uninterrupted sleep and wake up the next morning feeling rested and regenerated. However, this doesn't always work out the way we would like it to. Sometimes, it is not even a matter of not having enough time to sleep. It is about not being able to fall asleep. We have all had those restless nights when we go to bed, then toss and turn all night, and by the time we fall into a nice, deep sleep, it is already time to get up.

So let's take a look at ways we can help our bodies get the rest they need. I have a few things that I always try to do to help me to get a good night's sleep. One of the most important is that I do not drink any caffeine products. That includes pops, teas, and coffee, but can also include chocolate. A lot of people do not realize how much caffeine there is in many of our pops (as well as a great deal of salt). As I am sure that you know, caffeine is a stimulant and will make it hard for you to sleep. Caffeine can also interfere with hormones, and as any menopausal woman can tell you, it can intensify hot flashes.

One other important hint that works for me is that I try not to eat for at least three hours before I go to bed. If you eat shortly before you go to bed, it will often make it difficult for you to get a good night's sleep, and not only will it make you toss and turn, but it can also intensify heartburn or other digestion problems. Your body needs some time to digest the food you eat, so try and give yourself three hours of no food before bed.

Another technique that I use prior to sleep is to take some time to meditate and calm my mind. If you have had a lot of things happening in the day and you are worrying about those things, it is hard to turn your mind off, and that alone can make a good night's sleep elusive. I have developed some breathing exercises that I do before I go to bed and those, combined with focused meditation, help me to relax enough so that I fall asleep. I also will say positive mantras to myself so that I am going to sleep while programming good thoughts into my mind. I will often fall asleep while I am saying my positive mantras. Some people like to read before bed as a way to slow down. If this is something that works for you, I'd encourage you to read positive and uplifting things prior to bed to assist with sleeping. An engaging action novel or the latest Stephen King horror story may not be the best choices when you are struggling to get enough restful sleep.

If you choose to do some relaxing breathing, there are countless techniques, but I will share with you the one that I use. I concentrate on taking in a deep breath for a period of seven seconds, followed by a further period of seven seconds that I hold my breath, and then I spend another seven seconds exhaling. It is important to be inhaling for the full seven seconds, holding your breath for another full seven seconds, and exhaling for the final full seven seconds. This is a great way to fill your body with oxygen and help your mind and body to relax fully. While you are breathing in, you will want to try to rid your mind of any negative thoughts or worries and try not to think about anything except counting to seven during each of the three phases of breathing.

If you find your mind constantly bombarded with negativity, there are several tricks I have learned that help me to clear my mind of those negative thoughts. I will often replace the negative thought by saying a positive mantra to myself, such as, "I enjoy all the good that life has in store for me," or "I am so happy and grateful that I am healthy and my family is healthy." I will imagine that with each breath I inhale that I am bringing peace and tranquility into my body, mind, and spirit. When I exhale, I will imagine that I am releasing stress, conflict, and negative energy from my body. Positive energy in, negative energy out. This is a powerful tool to relax yourself and also to shift your mind into a positive vibration.

If I am trying to focus on weight loss, I will visualize that I am breathing in health and letting go of unwanted pounds. It is a good idea to start out by doing the counting for the seven second counts. Once you are in a calm and steady rhythm of breathing, then you can move toward positive visualizations. You may also want to use this time to do some positive self-talk or to visualize yourself being happy, healthy, and successful. Whenever a negative thought or worry comes into your mind, try to counteract the negative thought or worry with four positive statements. For example, "Everything is good. I am calm and relaxed. I feel good about myself. I am healthy and strong. I lose weight easily and effortlessly." You can tailor the thoughts to suit your life or your goals, but it is good to be ready with positive statements to counteract the negative thoughts or worries that may come into your mind.

Sometimes, if I have time before I go to sleep at night, I will put in a yoga CD and do a yoga routine before I go to bed. Most yoga routines take you through a series of stretches and end with a very relaxing breathing exercise. I find that I am ready to fall right asleep after doing one of these routines. Yoga is also a really good way to exercise. It is very low impact, so it is something that you can do regardless of your current level of fitness. Yoga helps you to stretch out the muscles in your body and helps you to breathe deeply to bring oxygen into your body. This relieves stress and keeps your body loose and free of tension.

Sleep Isn't the Only Way to Rest

While sleep is very important, sometimes we simply need to take a time-out from the hustle and bustle of our daily routines. There are ways you can do this throughout your day, and you would be surprised at how much of a difference short little breaks can help you to feel refreshed and get refocused in a positive way.

Some days can be more stressful than others. It seems that if you get started on the wrong foot, the rest of your day just keeps on going wrong. When you are having a day like this, try to take a mental break someplace quiet and get refocused to put yourself in a more positive vibration. Rather than go for lunch or a coffee break in a noisy cafeteria or lunchroom, try to find a quiet spot to do some deep breathing and to try to visualize the rest of your day getting better. See yourself as being very calm when dealing with whatever situation comes your way. See yourself as having patience and being able to tackle any situation with a positive and friendly attitude. It is a good idea to go for a walk on your break, breathe some fresh air, and mentally recharge your batteries. Sometimes a little bit of exercise is enough to kick you out of a stressful funk.

I would often put on my iPod and listen to relaxing music on the bus ride to or from work. Or if you drive, put in a nice CD to listen to as you drive into work or on the way home. Use your time wisely. Tune out the noise and tune in to your inner voice and inner guide, which is always there to guide you. Often in life, our inner voice is trying to guide us, but we get so caught up in the daily stresses that we never take the time to get quiet and reflect on where we are going or what we are doing. By taking time to get quiet, you can step back from your own life and situation and really take a good look at things. There may be a better direction for you to go, but if you never take the time to get quiet and think about things, you will never see what could be a better direction.

When stressful or upsetting situations happen, realize that this is a normal part of life and try to look for the blessings in all things that happen around you. Sometimes a situation will occur that you may originally think is negative, but often there will be a blessing or a lesson in the situation that will turn out to be for your benefit in the future. It is not always easy to see these blessings right away, but you will see them if you allow your mind to step away and view it objectively.

I remember when I was very young and foolish, I had a terrible boyfriend. He cheated on me, he was in trouble with the law, and he lied on a regular basis. I was young and short-sighted and would always take him back. He would spin some story and beg for forgiveness, and I wanted so badly for things to work out with him that I would always give him another chance and take him back, only to be hurt once again.

One day during an argument, he threw me down to the ground very hard. When I hit the ground, I dislocated my shoulder. I was so angry and upset that I filed police charges against this man, and the courts gave me a restraining order to keep him away from me. At the time this happened, I was devastated and felt so sorry for myself. I thought this was the worst thing that could ever have happened to me. This man went to jail for assaulting me, and I was awarded compensation through a criminal injuries compensation program. With the money I received, I was able to purchase my first home at a time when the real estate market was very affordable. Three years later, I sold the property and walked away with a large amount of money, which helped me to really get ahead in my life.

When I look back on this situation now, I realize that this assault was the best thing that could have happened to me. It helped me to rid myself of a lying, cheating, abusive boyfriend, and it also made it possible for me to be able to buy my first home. If the assault had not occurred, I would have endured a lot more grief by allowing him or others to treat me badly, and I also would never have been able to come up with enough money to buy my first home at such a great time. In hindsight, this was a huge blessing in my life, although I could not see it at the time.

Things often happen for a reason, and sometimes that reason is because we need a push to get going in the right direction in our lives. So look for the blessings and lessons that need to be learned in all situations. Everyone has bad things or stressful events happen to them during the course of their lives. People will die, people will get hurt, finances will be strained, and stressful situations are sure to occur. The best way that you can deal with these situations is to have the right attitude. Looking for the blessings and the lessons in these situations will help you to handle these situations better and make you a stronger person as a result.

The Power of Meditation

Meditation is a very powerful tool that is free to use. However, many of us fail to take advantage of the power of meditation. Meditation is defined as "deep, serious thought." It is about taking time to get quiet and reflect on life, or to simply clear your mind of all thoughts. It gives your brain a rest. It allows you to get in touch with your inner voice and spirit. It is a time to get focused on what you want out of life and to explore different ways to achieve your goals. It is a time for you to mentally recharge your batteries. It is a time to let go of stress and to allow yourself to completely relax.

Meditation is a healthy way to deal with anxiety and stress. Many people turn to drugs, alcohol, food, or other substances to deal with anxiety or stress in an unhealthy way. These methods really only exacerbate the problem and make you sick and unhealthy at the same time. By using substances to relax or deal with stress, you are only numbing yourself while putting chemicals into your body that will likely make you sick, overweight, or addicted to the substance. We all need time to ourselves, and meditation is a great way to get away from the stresses of life.

The practice of meditation is really very simple. There are two ways in which I meditate. One way is what I would call a focused meditation, and the second way is an unfocused meditation. They are both useful, but I use the different types of meditation for different reasons.

To get started, you will need to find a quiet and comfortable place to sit. As I live in the Rocky Mountains, I will often go out into nature to meditate when weather permits. However, most often I will meditate at home in my bedroom. If I am at home, and there are other people around, I will tell them that I do not want to be disturbed for the next 30 minutes. I will put a mat down on the carpet, or I will find a comfortable chair to sit in. You will want to be in a very comfortable position that you can stay in without moving for up to 30 minutes. For me, this is sitting against a wall with my legs crossed and my hands facing palms up and placed on each knee. Some people like to have their hands clasped in front of them. Find what position is most comfortable for you. When you are meditating, you will want to try to keep a good posture in your upper body so that you can open up your diaphragm and take in plenty of deep breaths. You will start by breathing in deeply and exhaling deeply. You want to be as still as possible. You may want to set an alarm or a timer for 30 minutes so you know when 30 minutes has elapsed and you don't get distracted wondering how long you have been meditating.

When I am doing a focused meditation, I am trying to put myself in a better frame of mind, or—as I like to call it—a better vibrational frequency. While I am doing a focused meditation, I am thinking about goals I would like to achieve in my life. If my goal is to have a thinner, healthier body, I will sometimes use a mantra I say to myself that will help me to draw in and focus my energy on achieving this goal. I might repeat a mantra like, "I am healthy and fit. Health and wellness are flowing to me continuously." I will try to visualize myself achieving the goal I desire, and I will try to really focus on what it would feel like to achieve my goal. I will imagine that I have achieved my goal, and I will try to get myself into a place of feeling what it is like to be where I want to be. This is a very powerful exercise. I believe that focusing intently on your goals helps to reprogram our subconscious mind to help us achieve our goals.

Sometimes, my goal is to simply let go of stress and anxiety and to get myself into a better frame of mind. I will simply visualize that I am breathing in peace and tranquility, and I am exhaling stress and anxiety. It is amazing how powerful this is to really let go of your stress and anxiety. You will find that when you are relaxed and at peace with yourself, then solutions to problems suddenly appear. You may find yourself inspired to move in a different direction that you never thought of before.

When I am doing an unfocused meditation, I simply want to clear my mind of all thoughts and simply breathe and remain quiet. It may be harder than you think to simply clear your mind of all conscious thoughts. This is a great way to get yourself in touch with your inner voice and spirit. I imagine that by clearing my mind of all conscious thought, I am then allowing the flow of inspiration, communication from the universe, my inner voice, and my spirit to flow toward me.

When you quiet your mind and stop consciously thinking, your subconscious mind can take over for a while, and this is when you will find that you will be inspired with an idea or a solution to a problem that may take you in the right direction you need to go. I don't consciously think about receiving inspiration; I just simply try to clear my mind of all conscious thought for a period of 15–30 minutes. I have simply noticed that when I do this, I usually am inspired shortly after the meditation in some way. I believe that giving your mind a rest allows you to get refreshed and perhaps have a fresh outlook on things. Try it and see what happens. You really have nothing to lose.

Stress Relief

Take a few minutes to think about how you currently handle stress. Do you eat when you are stressed or feeling anxious? Do you rant and rave and complain when you are stressed? Do you use drugs or alcohol when you are stressed? Do you go shopping or gambling when you are stressed? Or perhaps you smoke? Do you use stress as your excuse for these unhealthy habits?

I remember that if I used to have a really hard day, I would use the fact that I had a bad day to rationalize why I deserved to eat that hot fudge sundae or that extra large bag of potato chips. This was such an unhealthy way to handle my stress, but that is how I coped with my stress at that time in my life. In order to overcome this unhealthy way of dealing with my stress, I had to learn new and healthier ways of dealing with my stress to replace my bad habit of using food to handle it. I had to remove the unhealthy habit and replace it with a healthy one. Meditation is a great way to relieve stress in your life, but let's take a look at other ways in which we can relieve our stress or to simply make our lives less stressful.

One way to reduce your level of stress is to simply change your attitude about things. Do you find yourself getting angry or yelling a lot with little provocation? You can choose how you react to things. You can remain calm and even-tempered, regardless of the situation you are in. You can accept that it is normal for things to go wrong from time to time and that you will simply deal with what comes up in a calm and relaxed manner. Losing your temper, yelling, or complaining about your life is not going to solve anything. If you don't like your life, then change it. If you don't like your job, then let that motivate you to find a job that you do like. If you don't like the way that people are treating you, learn how to speak up for yourself or stop spending time with people who treat you poorly or don't uplift you. Spend your time focusing on looking for solutions and making things better, rather than spending your time whining and complaining about how bad things are in your life. One of my favorite sayings is, "Look for solutions, not excuses."

You also can control the type of people that you spend your time with. I think it is important to really pay attention to how you feel around different people, as people can be a major stressor. Some people will encourage you, uplift you, and want the best for you and others. Some people will make you laugh and feel joyful about life and will have a positive outlook on life. Other people, even though they may be family or friends, will make you feel uptight and anxious. They may make you feel inadequate and insecure. They may put you down and make you feel upset, discouraged, or negative about things. They may be predominantly focused on gossip, negative issues, and whining and complaining most of the time. These people may take advantage of you, which may make you feel hurt or insulted at times. Negative people can be a huge drain of your energy and cause you a lot of anxiety and stress.

So think about the people that you are spending your time with and ask yourself if they are the type of people you enjoy being around. Are they creating stress in your life, or are they uplifting you? You have a choice about whom you spend your time with, and if there are people in your life who cause you stress, avoid spending so much time with those people, or work at improving your relationship with those people so that it becomes more uplifting and less stressful.

We all will deal with stress at work at some point in our lives. This is normal. If you are having a bad day, make it a point to take a mental break from what is stressing you. If you can take a coffee break or a lunch break, get away from the workplace for your break and walk, stretch, breathe deeply, and just try to shift your thinking to something less negative. Try to look for what is right, rather than what is wrong. Try to focus on things in your life that make you feel happy and grateful. Try to make the best of the situation. Make it your deliberate intention that you will not let a stressful situation get the best of you. You will find that when you switch the way you think about things, the situation will improve.

Another great way to reduce stress is to plan ahead and to get yourself organized. Don't leave things to the last minute. Turn off your TV or computer and get to bed earlier so you can start your day earlier, which will give you plenty of time to get where you are going and to start your day off on the right foot. Plan your meals in advance. Set out your clothes for the next day the night before so that you won't be starting your day off in a panic. Plan a vacation or a fun activity to give yourself something good to look forward to. Plan time to exercise on a regular basis. Exercise is a great way to relieve stress, and it has the added benefit of making you healthier and fitter at the same time. By planning ahead and getting yourself organized, you will definitely reduce your stress, and you will feel happier and more in control of your life.

Balance is very important in our lives. All work and no play is not good for us. All play and no work isn't good, either. We need to have a balance with the activities we are doing and a balance with the people we spend our time with. Make some time to have some fun. Enjoy spending time with your children or family. Take time to spend some quality time with your spouse. Don't forget to nurture your relationships. Take time to be alone. Take time to socialize with friends. The point is to mix things up and give your life balance. Think of the things that enrich your life and try to get a balance between those things and your work and other responsibilities. As my father used to say, "Take time to stop and smell the roses." Life is not about the destination; it is about the journey.

CHAPTER 10

—Baby Steps 101—

One of the hardest things to do when making changes in your life is to just get started. We can read literally hundreds of books about how to eat right, lose weight, exercise, meditate, and reduce stress. But the hardest thing to do is to put your knowledge into action. How do we get started? We have all known things that we really should do or that we would really like to do, but we don't always do them. We procrastinate and find excuses. Why?

Taking that first step is sometimes harder than you think. In this chapter, I want to give you some real-life suggestions to get you to put your plan into action. If you know what to do and you never do it, then all that knowledge is worthless. I would like to help you to move from a place of procrastination to a place of action by following some simple steps to get you on your way. If you can follow these easy guidelines, you will be able to apply them to every goal you have in life, and you will experience one success after another.

Now let's talk about taking your first step. It is this first step that is the hardest, so if you can get it out of the way, you can start that forward motion that gives you the momentum to keep going.

You might be thinking that you have not achieved anything yet, but by simply reading this book, you have. The biggest mistake that people make when trying to achieve a big goal is the fact that they look at the end result as one goal that has to be accomplished in giant leaps. They try to determine every single step that they need to take to reach their goal before they even take the first step. Most people don't know exactly how they are going to get to the finish line, so they never take the first step to even try. This is what prevents most people from achieving success. If you can just take a small step that you know will move you in the direction of your goal, you are having success. Even if that step is a failure in your mind, you need to realize that any step that you take is a success.

Let me give you some examples so you can see what I mean. Imagine that you are inside a huge maze. It is dark inside, and you don't have a map or a guide to take you through the maze. You only have a candle that will light up a small area of the maze. So what do you do? You look at your current surroundings, and you take an inventory of your current situation. There is a solid wall behind you, so you know you cannot go backward and you must go forward. You have two directions you can go, left or right, but you are not sure which direction to take.

At this point you have three choices. You can stay where you are, you can go left, or you can go right. If you stay where you are, you can be sure that nothing will change. If you go left and you come to a dead end, then you have not failed; you have simply gained the knowledge that the correct way to go was right, so that knowledge helps you to move forward and make the correct choice the next time. Once you find your way back to the start, you can go to the right, with the knowledge that you are going in the right direction. The point that I am trying to make is that as long as you keep taking steps, you are going to get closer to your goal. You don't need to know the way to the end. You just have to keep taking steps, and you will eventually achieve what you want. When you stop taking steps, you stop making progress until you choose to begin again. There is no limit on the number of tries you get in life, and there is no reason not to begin again. So don't feel that you need to know every step you need to take in advance of taking a step. Just take a step!

Most people are so focused on the future and getting to the end result that they forget about what they can do right now, in the present moment. They forget about all the little steps in the middle, in between the first and last step, that get you to that great big goal. What you must focus on is breaking down that big goal into a bunch of much smaller steps that you can easily achieve right now. You need to acknowledge the fact that each step you take is a success. You don't get there with one step. You get there with thousands of steps, thousands of choices, and thousand of little successes that eventually get you to that big, long-term goal.

When I made the decision to lose weight and turn my life around, I did not know how I was going to get there. I simply knew that I was going to die trying, and I knew that I was going to do something—anything—to keep me moving in the right direction. Every step you take is a success, whether it is a successful step that moves you forward or a learning step that takes you left when you needed to go right. It doesn't matter—both types give you knowledge and move you forward.

If you want to make permanent and lasting changes in your life, you start by taking steps that will move you forward and making small changes that you can maintain. Please don't fall into the trap of going from one extreme to the other by implementing a drastic change you cannot maintain permanently. Below, I am going to list some small steps you can take to move you in the right direction to start making permanent change in your life.

Some of the steps will move you in the direction of becoming more happy and fulfilled, and some will move you in the direction of gaining better health, but they are all worthy, small steps anyone can accomplish.

As you look at the steps, you will see that you may have already taken some of those steps, or they may not apply to you, and that's fine. Just move on and take another. You may want to read through this list periodically and choose a step that you would like to work on. You can't do them all at once, so just start by working on one step that you think you can accomplish. You may notice that there are some steps you can take that are not on the list. So please feel free to add other steps, as this is just to get you started and can be expanded, depending on where you are on your journey toward optimum health and wellness.

101 Ideas or Steps for a Healthier and Happier Life.

1. Take some time to get yourself organized for success. Plan your meals in advance, and take the time to shop for the foods you will need for those meals so that you can make better choices.

2. Add a fruit or a vegetable to every meal.

3. Try to increase the meals you eat at home, or prepare at home, to avoid eating out as often.

4. If you have to eat out, try not to have fast food.

5. Try to eliminate or reduce the amount of pop or sugary drinks that you consume. Replace those drinks with water, herbal teas (without caffeine), or juice made from real fruit or vegetables (e.g., V8 juice)

6. Increase the amount of water you drink to at least eight glasses a day. You can count herbal tea in your intake of water, as long as there is no caffeine in it.

7. Reduce or eliminate caffeine from your diet. Coffee, tea, energy drinks, and many pops are full of caffeine.

8. Reduce or eliminate white flour and white rice from your diet. Choose whole grain flours instead of white flour for your bread products.

9. Learn more about the glycemic index and try to work on keeping your blood sugar levels steady. This will increase your energy levels and will help you to lose weight.

10. Try to reduce or eliminate the amount of dairy products that you eat and drink. Try soy milk, almond milk, or rice milk products instead of animal milk products.

11. If you drink alcohol, try to reduce the amount you drink.

12. Increase the amount of green vegetables you eat each day.

13. Choose organic foods when they are available and when you can afford them.

14. Avoid eating for at least two hours before you go to bed.

15. Try to increase the variety of foods you eat. Look for new recipes that can add a variety of foods to your diet. Eating the same foods over and over again can lead to food intolerances. The greater the variety of food you eat, the more balanced your nutrition will be, and the more interesting your food will be.

16. Take one hour every day for yourself. Use this time to rest, meditate, exercise, relax, or focus on goals that will make you happier and healthier.

17. When purchasing foods, avoid buying foods that have the first ingredient as sugar, glucose, fructose, or sucrose.

18. Avoid buying foods that contain lots of additives and chemicals.

19. Try to focus on eating foods that contain good nutrition and avoid eating junk foods, such as donuts, cookies, chips, ice cream, chocolates, candies, and pastries.

20. If you eat cereal, try to choose cereals that are lower in sugar and higher in fiber.

21. Try to find creative ways of adding vegetables to your meals. Add lettuce, tomatoes, cucumbers, sprouts, or other vegetables to sandwiches and add extra vegetables into soups, sauces, and stews.

22. If you need a snack, try some healthy alternatives. For example, unsalted nuts or seeds, such as almonds, pecans, Brazil nuts, pumpkin seeds, and sunflower seeds, veggies with hummus dip, fresh fruit, plain popcorn, or a big glass of water or herbal tea.

23. Replace the starchy item in your meal with a salad as often as possible (e.g., instead of potatoes, bread, rice, or pasta, add extra vegetables or a salad to your meal).

24. Eat a healthy breakfast each day. Try to make good glycemic index choices to keep your blood sugar levels stable.

25. Visit a health-food store and learn about and try eating some new products.

26. Avoid foods that are high in animal fats, trans-fatty acids, or hydrogenated fats, such as lard, butter, fatty meats, baked goods, potato chips, donuts, cookies, crackers, fried foods, processed cheese, margarine, mayonnaise, vegetable shortening, ice cream, and chocolate.

27. If you don't get enough calcium in your diet, supplement it with calcium pills.

28. Visit a naturopath to discuss your health.

29. Stop using laxatives; instead, find natural ways to keep yourself regular (e.g., drink plenty of water, eat prunes, and eat lots of fresh fruits and vegetables).

30. Avoid products that contain artificial sweeteners, such as Splenda, saccharin, and aspartame. Try using agave nectar, honey, or fruit purees or fruit juices as an alternative.

31. If you are taking prescription medications, do some research on your medication to educate yourself about possible side effects. Take time to look into other more natural ways of treating yourself.

32. Work on increasing your physical activity. Try to exercise for a minimum of 30 minutes at least three to four times a week.

33. Find a new sport or activity that is fun and you enjoy, which will get you more physically active. Try yoga, tennis, skiing, golfing, bike riding, dancing, skating, walking, swimming, rollerblading, hiking, fishing, basketball, hockey, soccer, baseball, bowling, or football.

34. Decrease the amount of time you spend in front of a television set or in front of a computer. Try to find other activities to do in your leisure time (e.g., gardening, walking, cleaning, exercising, spending quality time with family or friends, meditating, planning meals, or taking a class).

35. Try to reduce the amount of red meat that you eat. Try adding poultry, fish, legumes, quinoa, or other food items to your diet.

36. Try to eliminate or reduce the amount of smoked or highly refined meats that you eat, such as salami, bologna, wieners, pepperoni, and chicken nuggets.

37. Become more aware of the ingredients in the prepackaged foods that you eat. Avoid foods with high sugar, high sodium, artificial sweeteners, preservatives, MSG, additives, or hydrogenated fats.

38. Try using fresh foods you prepare yourself whenever possible.

39. Try to use healthier fats when cooking. Avoid butter, lard, or animal fats. Try using olive oil or vegetable oil.

40. Go to the doctor for a check-up to measure your blood pressure, cholesterol, blood sugar levels, and so forth. Have this done before you start making changes so you can see how your changes improve your health.

41. Become more aware of your relationship with food. Do you eat when you are emotional, upset, or angry? Do you view food as a way of comforting yourself? Do you use food as a coping mechanism? If you answered yes to any of these questions, consider joining a self-help group or getting some counseling to help you to develop a healthier relationship with food. Consider joining Overeaters Anonymous or other support groups to help you.

42. Try to become aware of what it feels like to be physically hungry and try to eat only when you are physically hungry. Avoid eating when you are stressed, anxious, upset, emotional, or depressed unless you are physically hungry. I usually decide that if my stomach is growling,

then I am physically hungry. Sometimes you think you are hungry when you are actually just thirsty, so try having a drink of water before deciding to snack.

43. Are you happy in your relationships? Take a good, hard look at the relationships you have in your life. Is there an equal balance of give-and-take in your relationships? Are you being uplifted by your relationships, or do they cause you a lot of conflict? Are your relationships harmonious or full of conflict? If you are unhappy in your relationships, try to find ways to make things work, or if you can't make it work, look at ending those relationships for ones that are uplifting, balanced, harmonious, and rewarding.

44. Are you happy with yourself? Do you like who you are? Are you listening to your inner guide and spirit? Take some time to reflect on who you are and make changes to help you to become the person you were meant to be. Instead of spending time criticizing others, take time to honestly take a look at yourself and what you need to change, rather than focusing on getting others to change.

45. Stop playing the blame game. Don't look to blame others for your unhappiness. Start taking responsibility for your own life and the quality of your life. If you are unhappy with your life, take charge and make a positive change.

46. Do you have a victim mentality? Are you always feeling sorry for yourself? Do you expect others to make you happy? Are you full of excuses about why you can't get what you want out of life? You need to look to yourself for happiness. Don't be a doormat, and don't be complacent about your life if you are unhappy. It is up

to you to make changes to move your life in the right direction to make yourself happy.

47. Are you a happy person? If not, take a look at how you view life. Do you expect the best out of life, or do you always expect the worst? Maybe you need to look at the world in a different way. Try approaching life with a more positive attitude. Look for the best in all situations.

48. Remember to take time to be grateful for all the good things you have in this life. Remember what is really important to you.

49. Are you abusing alcohol, drugs, or have some other addictive habit? Get help to deal with your addictions. Addictions can only lead to unhappiness. Using drugs and alcohol to forget about your troubles will only make matters worse. Don't be afraid to ask for help if you need it. Alcoholics Anonymous or Narcotics Anonymous are free support groups that can help you overcome addictions to alcohol or drugs.

50. Is there someone in your life who is struggling with addictions to drugs or alcohol? Consider joining a support group such as Al-Anon or Adult Children of Alcoholics to find out ways to help you deal with a loved one with addictions.

51. People and the relationships you have with them are very important in life. Reach out and be more open and loving to others. Try to nurture your relationships and be grateful for the people who love you. Don't take others for granted. Don't criticize and ridicule your children or spouse. Try to respect others and be understanding, loving, and helpful to them. Be patient.

Strive for harmony. Give and receive hugs when you or the one you love is having a hard day.

52. Are you a control freak? Are you always telling others how to lead their lives, even when they don't ask for your opinion? Do you enable others by always doing everything for them and not letting them find out how to do things on their own? Maybe you need to work on letting others be who they are and focus on yourself a bit more, and a bit less on others. Try to look after your own life and let others do the same. Allowing others to find their way helps them to grow stronger. Everyone makes mistakes, including you. We learn and grow from our mistakes.

53. If you think you are stressed out, find healthy ways of coping with your stress. Exercise and meditation are great ways to reduce your stress levels. Don't turn to alcohol, drugs, or food to reduce your stress. Don't waste your time getting angry and venting on others when you are stressed out. That will just make matters worse.

54. Try to look outside of the box. Be a leader, not a follower. Find creative ways to solve your problems and challenges in life. "Imagination is more important than knowledge," as Albert Einstein said.

55. Try to be as happy and as pleasant as you can as often as possible. People like happy, helpful, and pleasant people. Nobody likes a grumpy, pessimistic complainer. When you approach life with a better attitude, you will find that you will have better experiences in life.

56. Don't be a doormat. Set healthy boundaries for yourself. Treat others well, but also expect to be treated well in return. Mutual respect is a key ingredient in all relationships.

57. Take time to try new things in life. Try a new activity or a new food.

58. Educate yourself. Read a book, take a course, or listen to an audio book.

59. Uplift yourself. Listen to music, think happy thoughts, dance, fall in love, go after your dreams, or listen to a motivational speaker or CD.

60. Buy a journal and write down your thoughts and ideas. This is a good way to get focused on things in your life that concern you. This is also a good way to set goals or to look at the progress you are making in your life.

61. Try meditation. This is a great way to reduce stress, relax, or focus intently on things that matter the most to you.

62. Get control of your finances. If your finances are causing you stress, get help from a debt counselor or find ways to control your spending or increase your income. There are many ways to increase your income and reduce your spending. Here are a few ideas: Eat at home more often, take in a roommate, reduce money spent on entertainment, or have a garage sale to sell items that you no longer need. Downsize to a cheaper place to live or take in a roommate or renter. Sell your car and take the bus or walk or cycle to work. Carpool to work to save on gas. Get a part-time job or work toward getting a better-paying job. Consider talking to your banker to see if you can renegotiate your mortgage to reduce your interest rate or payments. Consider increasing your mortgage to pay down higher interest credit card debt if you have equity in your home. Reduce your spending on nonessential items.

63. Don't waste your time gossiping or criticizing others. Avoid being around negative people. Surround yourself with people who make you feel happy, positive, uplifted, and motivated. Try to spend your time encouraging and uplifting the people you spend your time with. Try to impact people in a positive way rather than a negative way.

64. How are your communication skills? Are you able to express yourself openly and honestly, or do you have a hard time saying no when you need to say no? Do you let others take advantage of your good nature? Are you assertive, or are you too aggressive or too passive? Work on improving your communication skills to help you improve your relationships with others. You can do this by reading a book, taking a course, or hiring a coach or a counselor.

65. If you are a parent, try to love and encourage your child. Avoid being critical and judgmental. Lead by example. If you want your child to respect you, learn how to treat your child with respect also. Don't be afraid to hug your children and tell them how much you love them. If you had a bad experience as a child growing up, try to learn from that experience and give your child a better experience.

66. Remember to try to look for the good in all circumstances and remember to look for the lessons in life. Sometimes our greatest achievements come from our greatest disappointments or tragedies in life.

67. Work on improving your self-esteem and your appearance. Do something to make you look and feel better about yourself. Get a haircut, get rid of the gray hair by dyeing it, put on some makeup, shave your

stubble, buy some new clothes, take pride in your appearance by paying a bit more attention to your grooming habits, such as brushing your teeth, shaving your face, shaving your legs, trimming/painting your finger/toenails, fixing up your hair, showering regularly, and using deodorant, aftershave or perfume to smell good. When you look and smell good, you will feel good!

68. If you love someone, let them know. Don't let your fear of rejection allow you to miss an opportunity. Feel the fear and do it anyway.

69. Try to approach life with a joy-based mentality rather than a fear-based mentality. Instead of focusing on what might go wrong, focus on what might go right.

70. Forgiveness is about letting go of all the negative emotions and simply forgiving someone for something that they may have done to you. Remember that everyone makes mistakes. Some of us learn from our mistakes and become better people as a result of the mistakes we have made. Some of us take longer to learn than others. Learn to forgive. Let go of your anger, hatred, and rage. It is poisoning you to have those negative emotions inside of you. You will feel relieved to let go of those negative emotions. Forgiveness is not about condoning the behavior of the person who has wronged you. Forgiveness is about letting go of the negativity that can consume you and make you unhappy. Forgiving allows you to move on with your life in a positive direction, and it gives you the opportunity to learn and understand from the experience.

71. Get plenty of sleep and work on improving your quality of sleep. If you have a hard time sleeping, look into ways

of helping yourself relax naturally before you go to sleep. Here are a few suggestions to help you sleep better: Try not to eat at least two to three hours before going to sleep, avoid using caffeine products, exercise regularly, and meditate or read before going to sleep. Get earplugs if it is too noisy for you to sleep. Buy a better mattress or pillow if you are uncomfortable when you sleep.

72. Quit smoking.

73. If you have lost weight or are losing weight, make sure to take pictures of yourself through the process of losing weight and take time to look at them. It is important to mentally readjust your internal image of yourself so that it matches your external image. If you are thin but still view yourself as a fat person, you are going to have a hard time maintaining your weight loss. Get used to seeing yourself as a happy, thin, and healthy person. You should try to put this image of yourself in your mind even before you lose the weight. Visualize yourself as you would like to be.

74. Use sunscreen when you are out in the sun.

75. Try to improve your education to assist you in getting a better job or career.

76. How is your work environment? If you are truly unhappy in your work environment, look for another job or work at starting up your own business or educating yourself so that you can get a better job.

77. Don't waste your time looking for excuses to justify why you are not getting to where you want to be. Instead, focus your time looking for solutions and ways to get you to where you want to be.

78. Forgive yourself for mistakes you have made in the past. Remember that no man or woman is defined by one

moment in their life. We are all growing and learning.
Learn from the past, and then leave it behind and move
in a better direction in the future.

79. Stop dieting! You are not on a diet. You are simply
making small permanent changes that will move you
in a healthier direction in your life. It is not the end of
the world if you occasionally make an unhealthy choice.
You simply try to make better choices most of the time
and get adjusted to healthier ways of living your life that
are manageable for you.

80. Watch movies or listen to audio CDs that motivate and
uplift you. If you can afford it, hire a coach to help you
with weight loss or lifestyle changes.

81. Live with a clean conscience. Try to treat others well and
feel good about who you are and the impact that you are
having in the world. Be charitable and loving to others.
We are all on this earth together and we should try to
help and encourage others rather than hurt and ridicule
each other.

82. If you have the time and resources to have a pet, then
consider getting one. Animals are great stress reducers.
If you have a dog, it will encourage you to get out and
walk with your dog. If you decide to get a pet, make
sure that you are committed to caring for that animal
financially, emotionally, and physically. Pets take time.
They need to be fed, cleaned, played with, and provided
with shelter. Most of all, they need love and affection.
Relationships with pets can be very rewarding. Just
make sure you are committed to giving the time, money,
and attention needed to properly love and care for your
pet.

83. Spend 15 minutes in the morning and an additional 15 minutes at night doing some positive visualization or positive self-talk. Positive visualization is intently focusing on what you want to manifest in your life. Positive self-talk is complimenting yourself, focusing on all the things you like about yourself, and imagining yourself as you would like to be.

84. Whenever someone puts you down or insults you, or whenever you put yourself down, you must counteract the negative statement immediately with four positive statements about yourself. For example: Insult: "How could you be so stupid?" Positive statements: "I am an intelligent person, I work hard to make a good home for my family, I am a beautiful person on the inside and a beautiful person on the outside, and I am very thoughtful and caring."

85. If you fall down or fail, get up, dust yourself off, learn from your failure, and try, try again.

86. Develop a network of family and/or friends that is supportive and encouraging to you to help keep you on track and get you through the tough days, as well as to celebrate your successes along the way.

87. Struggling with a goal? Hire a coach or a counselor, attend a motivational seminar, or buy a motivational book. Spend a little money to get the help that you need. Invest in yourself. You are worth it!

88. Enjoy sex in a healthy and safe manner. Sex is a great way to relieve stress and to bond with the person you love.

89. Don't sweat the small stuff. Relax and try not to worry or get yourself stressed out about little things that won't matter a year from now. Remember what is really

important out of life. If you only had a week to live, would the item that you are now stressing out about really matter? If not, take a deep breath and just let it go.

90. Make sure to take time for yourself. Take care of yourself first. If you don't look after yourself, you won't be able to look after anyone else.

91. Practice how to take a compliment without discounting it.

92. Help others when you can, and be willing to accept help from others.

93. No one knows you better than you! Listen to your inner voice and let it guide you.

94. Take time to stop and smell the roses. Take time to slow down and enjoy the moment you are in right now. Many people get so focused on getting somewhere that they never stop to enjoy themselves in the current moment. Remember that life is about the journey, not about the destination.

95. Love people; use money. Many people love money and use people. Money is worthless if you have nobody to share it with you. While we all need to make enough money to survive and pay our bills, don't let your pursuit for the almighty dollar prevent you from enjoying the more important things in life, like family, friends, your health, fun experiences, and a self-image that allows you to feel good about yourself as a person.

96. Set realistic goals for yourself. Don't try to do everything at once. Pick something that you would like to accomplish and work on that goal. It is better to set small goals and achieve them, rather than repeatedly fail at unrealistic goals.

97. If you make a mistake, or if you have wronged someone, have the courage to look at your mistakes, admit them, apologize, and try to make amends. At the very least, learn from your mistakes. We all make them.

98. Try to be true to yourself and others. Let down your guard, set aside your image, and let the real you shine through. Be your genuine and true self. Say what you mean and mean what you say. Don't pretend to be something that you are not.

99. Take time to find a life partner to share your life with. On your search for your life partner, it is wise to pay less attention to physical attributes and more attention to the beauty within. If you already have a life partner, take time to nurture your relationship and your partner, and take time to be grateful for your relationship.

100. Do something nice for someone else anonymously. If anyone finds out that you did it, then it doesn't count. This is about giving to someone else without the expectation of anything in return. It will make you feel good, and it will also make the person you did something nice for feel good, as well.

101. Make a difference. When you leave this world, will the world be a better place in some way because of your existence? Try to leave a positive ripple in the world and in the lives of the people you touch.

CHAPTER 11

—Real People, Real World—

Every person who reads this book is going to be at a different place. Some of you may know how to cook, and others may not. Some of you already have exercise as part of your life, and others will view exercise with a very negative attitude. We all have different eating habits, and some of them are going to be better than others. So if you are able to cook, do not cringe at the thought of doing some exercise, and have fairly good eating habits, you are starting far ahead of many others. Your place of starting is going to be much different from someone who never cooks, never exercises, and who eats mostly fast food or highly processed foods.

I think it is also important to look at where your starting point is in regard to your mental attitude and well-being. Some of you are happy, while others may be angry, depressed, hopeless, full of excuses, or struggling in a bad relationship. Some of you may have a positive outlook on life, while others may have a negative attitude or feel that life is painful and depressing. We all are at different levels of self-esteem. Many of us are lonely. Some of us have already done some work on ourselves by reading self-help books or getting help from a counselor, while others don't even know where to begin to implement changes.

This book is not just about losing weight. This book is about finding health and happiness and leading a joyful and fulfilling life. There are plenty of thin people out there who are unhealthy and unhappy, and there are many people who are overweight but are healthier and happier than people who are thin. So think about where your starting point is and try to follow some of the guidelines in this book to move you to a happier and healthier place in your life. It doesn't happen overnight, but it will happen if you keep taking steps in the right direction.

Nobody in this world is perfect. I will be the first person to admit that I am not perfect. I don't eat perfectly all the time, and I have good times and bad times, just like anyone else. I don't have a perfect body, mind, or spirit. I am human, just like you are. We are always growing and changing. What I can tell you for sure is that your life can get better than it is right now. It will never be perfect, but it can and will be much better if you start to move yourself in a different direction and try to incorporate some of the ideas and suggestions in this book. You have nothing to lose. It is never too late to start, no matter where you begin. Things will only get better.

Here are a few suggestions to help you along your way.

1. Buy a Notebook and a Pen

I have found it very helpful to simply write things down in a notebook. Over the years, I have written down different thoughts and ideas I have had about my health and wellness along the way. I made it a point to note how I was feeling, what my clothes size was, my weight, my struggles, and my successes along the way. It was almost like a scientist chronicling his experiments. I would indicate different diets I tried along the way, and what worked and what didn't. I wrote about my thoughts and ideas, my hopes, my goals, and my dreams. Sometimes you don't realize how much progress you are making in life. I have found it very interesting to go back and read through my notes I have made over the years to see how much progress I have made mentally, physically, and emotionally. There was never really one big step I took that really made the difference. It was all of the little steps along the way that added up to the big changes in my life. So it is really helpful to document your journey, and perhaps you will one day get to write about your success story also.

I also make it a point to write down all of the things that I am grateful for in my life in my journal. It helps me to keep my mind focused on the good things in my life, rather than focusing on fears and negativity. Try to come up with at least 20 things that you are grateful for in your life.

Here are a few suggestions of things that you might be grateful for: You live in a free country, you have access to health care, you have food to eat , you have a home and a bed to sleep in, you have people who love and care about you, you have clothes to wear, you can walk, you can breathe fresh air, you can read, you can write, you have a brain that gives you the ability to learn and to make choices that will enable you to have a better life, and you have the free will to live your life any way that you choose.

2. Make a Plan, Set Some Goals, and Get Organized

Take an honest look at where you are in your life and try to see the ways in which you could make changes that will last. Plan ahead to succeed. Look at the reasons why you have not succeeded in the past and look for solutions to help you to succeed.

In a perfect world, we would always have the time and energy to exercise, cook healthy meals, and get plenty of rest. However, our world is not always perfect, and life can get very busy at times, so I wanted to leave you with a few tips and suggestions to help you get yourself organized for success.

To help me to succeed in eating healthier, I try to plan my meals in advance. I try to have healthy choices on hand so that I can grab something in a hurry and eat it on the way if I am running late. On the day before I return to work after my weekend, I will boil some eggs to have ready for a quick snack of protein in the morning. I make sure that I go shopping so that I have some fresh fruit and veggies in the fridge. I always have soy milk in the fridge. I also stock up my freezer with frozen fruits, vegetables, and meats.

I don't always have time to cook, so if I make a meal, I will make extra portions and put them in the freezer to eat on another day when I don't have as much time.

I always keep ready-to-eat salads in the fridge. The lettuce has already been washed, so all I have to do is throw the salad mix on a plate, add a cucumber or tomato and some dressing, and I am ready to eat. I will sometimes cook up a few chicken breasts at the start of the week and put them in the fridge so that they are ready to quickly slice up and throw onto a salad for some quick protein.

Look at your current schedule and try to find ways to change your routine around to give you more chances to succeed. Watching TV or surfing the Internet is a big time waster. Try to change your routine around to make things work for you. Remember to get your priorities right. Is it more important to watch TV, or is it more important to plan ahead for success?

3. Learn How to Cook

There are a lot of people out there who simply don't know how to cook. By not being able to cook, you will spend a lot more money on food that is less healthy for you than if you made it at home. You don't have to get really fancy or anything to be able to prepare meals at home. Anyone can boil an egg or make a sandwich or a salad at home. You just need to buy a couple of pots and pans, and you can be cooking before you know it. If you really don't know how to cook, ask a friend or family member for help. Go on the Internet or go to the library to look up cooking techniques and recipes. If you already know how to cook, try some new recipes to keep your meals healthy and interesting. You should also make it a point to ease yourself into eating new foods that you don't normally eat. If you don't like vegetables, then try adding butter or a sauce to them until you get used to eating vegetables. I think it is better to eat broccoli that is covered with butter or to eat fresh vegetables with a dip than it is to never eat vegetables at all.

Remember that this is about taking baby steps. You have to be able to live with your changes on a permanent basis. You don't have to be perfect at this. Just slowly move yourself in a better direction. Once you get used to eating vegetables, you can try to eat them with less sauces and butters. But you can worry about that later. Just take that first step. The same goes for adding fish into your diet. A lot of people never eat fish. If you really don't like eating fish, just try having fish and chips once a week. As you get used to that, you can try having the fish with a salad, and then perhaps try and have the fish pan-fried without batter. It takes time to get used to eating differently, so don't worry about being perfect. Just start to implement changes that you can live with.

4. Find a Way to Fit Exercise into Your Life on a Regular Basis

I have written an entire chapter in this book about exercise, so I won't go into too much detail about exercise again. However, I just want to remind you that exercise is a critical part of becoming healthier. If you don't like exercise, you are not alone. Many of us have a very negative view about exercise because it can be hard work. I used to detest exercise. However, my attitude has changed, and I have learned to really enjoy it and look forward to it. I would just suggest that you take baby steps with regard to exercise. Make small changes like taking the stairs instead of taking the elevator sometimes, or getting off the bus one stop earlier and walking a bit of the way. Perhaps you can just turn on the music at home and exercise or dance to a bit of music. If you are really out of shape, you can start by just doing some stretching or arm movements to get yourself moving a little bit more than you are right now. The main point is to do something. You have to get your body moving if you want to get in shape.

The Power of Now

A lot has changed in my life since that day when I cried at my kitchen table and felt hopeless and alone. I can't fully explain to you how good it feels to have made such a big transformation in my life, but I do want to try my best to describe it to you so you can start to feel within yourself that whatever you desire can be achieved. I want to help you to find the way to health and happiness. I want to be a role model, to show you and others that change is possible. If I can do it, you can do it also. If you are unhappy with your life right now, you need to know that a better life awaits you. You can have the life that you have always wanted. You don't have to stay where you are right now. You are capable of change.

So how does it feel for me to have turned my life around? It feels really good to be at a healthy weight and to feel happy in my life. Life is joyful for me. I have a lot to be grateful for. I went from being overweight, full of aches and pains, and very depressed and hopeless to someone who is healthy and fit, free from aches and pains, and happy and excited about life. I am happy with myself. I am open and loving toward others. I feel good about the person that I have become, and I know that my struggles were necessary for me to grow and to evolve into the person that I have become. I feel so proud of myself for not giving up and for having the courage and belief in myself to go after my dream of health and happiness.

I have regained my health. I am no longer obese. I feel healthy and strong. I feel energetic and uplifted. I exercise regularly for an hour or longer at least four to six times a week. I look forward to exercise. I feel great when I exercise. I enjoy keeping active and fit. I realize how much I benefit from going to the gym. It helps me to reduce stress. Going to the gym helps me to have a healthy and strong body, and it is a way to meet and socialize with others who are in the same mindset as me when it comes to fitness.

It feels great to be in good physical shape and to enjoy the activities that I love and that are fun and exciting to me. I stopped trying to impress others, and I work now to impress myself. I have found out who I truly am. I am happy with that person. She is beautiful on the inside and beautiful on the outside. I like the person I have become, and I feel good about myself.

My children are happy and healthy and feeling positive about their future. They are excited about life, and they are looking forward to their future. They know what is important in life. I have tried to let my children be who they are and to love them unconditionally. I encourage them, and I always try to be a positive role model in their lives. I have educated my children about food and nutrition to help them make the best choices. I have shown them that exercise can really make you feel good. I am happy to see them both enjoying exercise and eating healthier.

I have ended my unhappy marriage, and I am in a loving relationship with a wonderful man who treats me the way I have always wanted to be treated. I know now that I had to learn to love myself and to be happy on my own before I could truly be happy with someone else. I have learned to openly accept love and compliments and to realize that I am worthy and deserving of love. I was always good at nurturing and giving to others. However, I realize now that I had to learn how to accept love and nurturing from another person. That was very hard for me because it was unfamiliar to me to be loved and nurtured.

Life can be stressful for all of us at times. I have learned healthier ways of dealing with that stress. I realize the benefit of meditation and relaxation. I realize how important it is to try to be calm when things don't always work out the way that I would like. Some days, I handle my stress better than on other days. I know that getting angry or looking to place blame never solves anything. I have learned to be more understanding of others and to realize that none of us are perfect. We all make mistakes, and it is always better to focus on dealing with ways to make things better, rather than spend any of my time complaining or getting angry about things.

I find that with the right attitude, even when things go wrong, it all works out in the end. I will often ask myself, "Will this really matter five years from now?" or, "I am going to try and look for the good in this circumstance." Even if I make a bad choice or a wrong turn, I know that I am always moving in the right direction, and it is normal to have little bumps along the way.

I am not fanatical about my eating. I don't follow any set diet plan. I simply try to make the best choices most of the time. I will indulge from time to time in alcohol, treats, and foods that

I know are not good for me. I have good days and bad days, just like everyone else. I get off track from time to time, but I know how to get back on track. I have a different attitude and a different way of looking at life. I do not feel like I am on a diet. I have just slowly adjusted my preferences for what I like to eat. As I educated myself about the effect that some foods were having on me, I began to choose to avoid those foods. I know that I control my energy levels and my moods by what I put into my body.

I educated myself about blood sugar levels, insulin, and the effect that different foods have on my blood sugar. I learned how to keep my blood sugar level stable by learning about the glycemic index. I know controlling my blood sugar levels keeps me feeling energetic, and it has virtually stopped my moodiness. I understand that my moodiness came from the fluctuations in my blood sugar levels. It is my preference to eat what makes me feel energetic, uplifted, and happy.

I learned about healing myself naturally. I have removed the amount of chemicals I put into my body that were contained in prescription drugs, junk food, over-the-counter medicines, alcohol, and coffee. I have educated myself about naturopathic ways of healing. I have learned to eat so that I keep my digestive system moving regularly. If constipation occurs, I drink as much water as possible, and I keep drinking it until my digestive system gets moving. I have learned to pay attention to the signals and cues that my body is giving me all the time to let me know when things are going well or not so well.

I choose to associate with positive, uplifting people, and I choose to be positive and uplifting to others. I changed my attitude. I stopped whining and complaining. I am taking time to enjoy the simpler things in life. I am grateful for the wonderful family and friends I have in my life. I make it a point to remember to be grateful for all the good things that I have in my life. I try to be respectful and kind to others. I look forward to trying new things in my life. I have learned to look at life with a joy-based mentality rather than a fear-based mentality. I would rather focus on what might go right instead of what might go wrong. I don't let fear paralyze me from moving forward.

I spend a lot of my time with a smile on my face. I learned to be myself and feel good about who I am. I think it is important for all of us to work at finding our joy vibe. I make it a habit to be happy and positive. I choose to be friendly and helpful. I continue to educate myself about ways to improve my health and well-being. I have learned to be someone who is in control of her life. I have learned to actively live my life. I stopped procrastinating, and I just got on with it. I learned how to love myself and others. I consciously made it my deliberate intention to have a positive impact on our world. I stopped being a victim. I stopped blaming others for my unhappiness. I learned to stop looking for excuses and to look for solutions instead. I learned to look to myself for my happiness, rather than to expect others to make me happy.

This is my philosophy; we all have the right to believe what we want to believe. You can believe what you want to believe. This is what I choose to believe:

- **I have the knowledge to make my life better.**
- **My knowledge gives me the power to change.**
- **The changes I make allow me to have power over my own destiny.**
- **I choose my destiny to be what I want for myself, and I will diligently move forward by taking one step at a time, knowing that every step I take is improving my life on a steady and sustained level throughout my entire life.**
- **So what do I choose for my life?**
- **I choose to be happy.**

- I choose to love and accept myself and others for who they truly are, and I know that everything will be okay.
- I choose to take responsibility for my own happiness.
- I choose to look for what is right in my life, rather than what is wrong.
- I choose to eat and drink in ways that make me feel good and full of energy.
- I choose to move and exercise my body, to keep my muscles and bones strong.
- I choose to nurture my mind and spirit by continuing to learn, by getting adequate sleep and rest, by letting go of the past by forgiving myself and others, by having fun, by loving others, by nurturing my relationships with others, and by being positive and uplifting toward others.
- What do I know about my life?
- I know that choosing to eat healthy and to exercise regularly gives me the ability to control the way that I look and the way that I feel.
- I know that by keeping my body full of good nutrition, my immune system will be stronger, I will not get sick as often, and I will decrease the risk of getting cancer, heart disease, stroke, diabetes, arthritis, and other diseases and illnesses.
- I know that how I eat and how much I exercise directly affects the way that I look and feel by reducing body fat, improving my complexion, having less bloating and constipation, lower blood pressure, better joint health, more vibrant and healthy-looking eyes, nice healthy teeth and gums, strong, shiny hair, stronger fingernails, more youthful-looking skin, less acne and skin rashes, improved

sex life, improved mental functioning and emotional well being, less mood swings, and less stress on my vital organs because they are not being overloaded with avoidable chemicals, toxins, preservatives, hormones, antibiotics, stimulants, drugs, and unhealthy foods and drugs.

I changed my life one small step at a time. I stopped procrastinating, and I just decided to start to take small steps toward my goals.

One of the best things you can do to help yourself is to learn to act right now. Let go of the past and do what you can do right now in this moment to make a positive change in your life. There is a way to achieve your goals if you are willing to believe in yourself more and are willing to have an open mind to making changes. Keep focused on what you want and keep working toward your goals. If you can take action today, then just do it.

I have worked hard and diligently toward making small, steady changes in my life that have resulted in a huge transformation in my body, mind, and spirit. The change was not overnight, and I am still keeping an open mind to continue to make changes and to adjust my attitudes and habits as I learn more. I don't know all of the answers. I am continuing to learn and grow, just like everyone else. I firmly believe that when you think you know all of the answers, you stop learning. I don't ever want to stop learning. I hope you will learn some things from this book that will help you through your journey in this life. If that happens, then I have succeeded in my purpose for writing this book and sharing my story with you.

So take the first step. Not later, not tomorrow, but right now! Now it is up to you. You can stay at the start of your maze and not ever make a move, or you can take a step right now, knowing that any step is better than never taking a step. Make a simple decision that you will make one small change in your life within the next week. I hope you will find health and true happiness. Your future self thanks your current self for having the courage to take the next step to move you in the right direction. Good luck!

LaVergne, TN USA
25 August 2010
194506LV00004B/6/P